Endocrinology

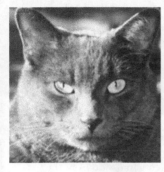

for the Small Animal Practitioner

David L. Panciera, DVM, MS
Diplomate ACVIM
(small animal internal medicine)
Professor
Virginia-Maryland Regional College of
Veterinary Medicine
Department of Small Animal
Clinical Sciences
Virginia Tech

Anthony P. Carr, Dr. med. vet.
Diplomate ACVIM
(small animal internal medicine)
Associate Professor
Small Animal Clinical Sciences
Western College of Veterinary Medicine
University of Saskatchewan

T0132678

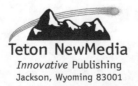

Teton NewMedia
Innovative Publishing
Jackson, Wyoming 83001

Executive Editor: Carroll C. Cann
Development Editor: Susan L. Hunsberger
Art Director: Sue Haun www.fiftysixforty.com
Production Manager: Mike Albiniak www.fiftysixforty.com

Teton NewMedia
P.O. Box 4833
Jackson, WY 83001
1-888-770-3165
www.tetonnm.com

PRINTED IN THE UNITED STATES OF AMERICA

ISBN # 1-893441-14-8

Print number 5 4 3 2 1

Library of Congress Cataloging-in-Publication Data

Panciera, David.
    Endocrinology for the small animal practitioner / David Panciera, Anthony B. Carr
    p. cm. – – (Made easy series)
    Includes bibliographical references (p.).
    ISBN 1–893441–14–8
        1. Veterinary endocrinology. I. Carr, Anthony P., 1960 – II. Title. III. Made easy series
    (Jackson, Wyo.)
    SF768.3P36 2005
    636.089'64 – – dc22

2005048546

Dedication

To Greta, Joe, and Mike, for their love, patience, and support.
David L. Panciera

To my mentors David and Richard, your guidance on my way to becoming an internist made a world of difference. I also dedicate this book to my family, the true meaning of life.
Anthony P. Carr

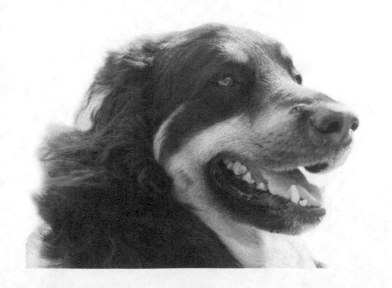

Preface

The diagnosis and management of endocrine disorders can be challenging. Clinical signs may be nonspecific and test results can be influenced by factors unrelated to the primary disease process. Treatment can also be demanding, as therapy must be individualized to account for differences in disease severity, etiology, and response to medication.

This book is an attempt to provide an organized and concise overview of endocrinology for practicing veterinarians. It was our goal to emphasize points that are clinically relevant and thereby provide practical guidelines for diagnosing and treating endocrine disorders. We made every effort to point out potential pitfalls in diagnosis and therapy where appropriate. Because of the considerable variation among animals with the same disease, this text is meant to act as a guide to diagnostic and therapeutic options rather than a cookbook where the approach to each disorder is strictly adhered to.

We hope this text will be helpful to you and that you will have it close by for frequent use. Although patients with endocrine disease can be very complex and frustrating, it can be a gratifying experience to finally piece the puzzle together and get the patient on the road to recovery.

David L. Panciera
Anthony P. Carr

Table of Contents

Section 1 Polydipsia and Polyuria

Section 2 Disorders of Growth Hormone

Section 3 Hypothyroidism

Section 4 Hyperthyroidism

Section 5 Hyperadrenocorticism

Section 6 Hypoadrenocorticism

Section 7 Hyperaldosteronism

Section 8 Pheochromocytoma

Section 9 Diabetes Mellitus

Section 10 Diabetic Ketoacidosis

Section 11 Hypoglycemia

Section 12 Hypercalcemia

Section 13 Hypocalcemia

Appendices

Index

Problem Index

A   = hypoadrenocorticism
ALDO   = hyperaldosteronism
C   = hyperadrenocorticism
D   = diabetes mellitus and
               diabetic ketoacidosis
DI   = diabetes insipidus
G   = growth hormone excess
G-   = growth hormone
               deficiency
HC   = hypocalcemia
HiC   = hypercalcemia
HG   = hypoglycemia
HT   = hyperthyroid
P   = pheochromocytoma
T   = hypothyroid

Abdominal mass   P, C, HG
Adrenal gland mass   C, P, ALDO
Alopecia   C, G-, T, HT
Anemia (non-regenerative)   A, T
Anorexia   HT, D, HC, HiC, A
Ascites or hemoabdomen   P
Ataxia   T, HG, D
Azotemia   A, G, HT, HiC
Bradycardia   A, T
Calcinosis cutis   C
Cataract   D, HC
Collapse   P, A, HG, HC
Comedones   C
Diarrhea   A, HT, HiC
Distended abdomen   C
Dwarfism, proportionate   G-

Dwarfism, disproportionate	T
Elevated liver enzymes	C, G, HT, D
Enlarged head	G
Enlarged tongue	G, T
Erythrocytosis	G, HT, C
Facial nerve paralysis	T
Facial rubbing	HC
Galactorrhea	T
Glycosuria	G, D
Head Tilt	T
Heart murmur	G, HT, ALDO
Hepatomegaly	C, D, G
Hyperactivity	HT
Hypercalcemia	A, HiC
Hypercholesterolemia	C, G, T, D
Hyperglycemia	G, D, C
Hyperkalemia	A
Hypernatremia	ALDO, DI
Hypertension	C, P, HT, ALDO
Hyperthermia	HC
Hypoalbuminemia	A
Hypoglycemia	HG, A
Hypokalemia	ALDO, HT, D
Hyponatremia	A, T, DI
Hyporeflexia	T
Hypothermia	T
Increased body weight without obesity	G
Increased nail growth	HT
Infertility	T
Insulin resistance	G, C, HT, T, D
Isosthenuria or hyposthenuria	A, C, G, HT, DI, HiC
Lameness, DJD	G
Lethargy	A, T, HiC
Melena	A
Muscle wasting	C, T, HT

Muffled heart sounds	T
Nystagmus	T
Obesity	C, T, D
Organomegaly (liver, kidneys, heart)	G
Otitis Externa	T
Panting or dyspnea	C, P, HT, HC
Peripheral neuropathy	D, T, HG
Polydipsia	A, C, G, P, HT, DI, ALDO, D, HiC
Polyphagia	C, G, HT, D, HG
Polyuria	A, C, G, P, HT, DI, ALDO, D, HiC
Prognathia	G
Proteinuria	G, C
Pyoderma	T, C
Seborrhea	T, HT
Seizures	HC, HG, HiC
Stridor	G
Stiff gait	HC
Stupor, Coma	T, HG
Tachyarrhythmias	P, HT
Tetany	HC
Thin skin	C
Tremors, Twitching	HC, HG, HiC
Urinary tract infection	C, D, HiC
Urolithiasis	HiC, C
Vomiting	A, P, HT, HiC
Weak pulse	T, A
Weakness	A, P, T, HT, ALDO, HC, HiC
Weight loss	HT, ALDO, D, A
Widened interdental spaces	G
Ventral flexion of the neck	HT, ALDO

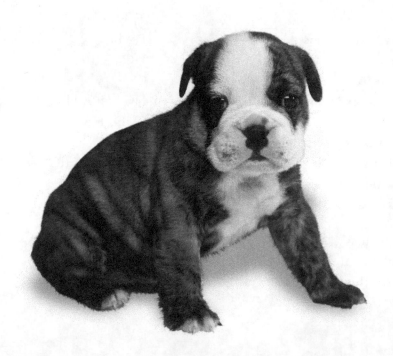

Section 1

Polyuria and Polydipsia

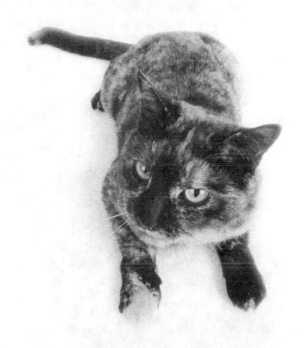

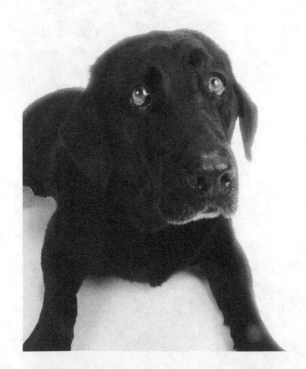

Introduction

The goals of this book is to provide a practical and succinct presentation of clinical endocrinology that will allow the practitioner to effectively diagnose and treat endocrine disorders. A problem index is provided that is keyed to each disorder as an aid for differential diagnosis. We hope that the descriptions of the diagnostic and therapeutic protocols will translate directly into patient management in your practice.

Some Helpful Hints

The following icons are used in this book to indicate important concepts:

✓   Routine. This feature is routine, something you should know.

♥   Important. This concept strikes at the heart of the matter.

🔑   Key. This concept is a key one and is necessary for full understanding.

💣   Something serious will happen if you don't remember this, possibly resulting in the loss of both patient and client.

✋   Stop. This doesn't look important but it can really make a difference.

Overview

♥ Polydipsia is defined as water consumption in excess of 100 ml/kg/day in a dog or cat, although most small animals drink less than 60 ml/kg/day.

♥ On repeated urine samples, a specific gravity above 1.030 rules out ongoing PU/PD while persistently low urine SG (<1.015) confirms PU/PD.

✔ There are numerous endocrine and non-endocrine causes of polyuria and polydipsia (PU/PD).

✔ By obtaining a thorough history, physical examination, and minimum data base most cases can be readily diagnosed.

♥ Causes of Polyuria and Polydipsia

Diabetes mellitus

Renal failure

Hyperadrenocorticism

Hypercalcemia

Hyperthyroidism

Pyometra

Post-obstructive diuresis

Hepatic failure

Pyelonephritis

Hypoadrenocorticism

Iatrogenic

Acromegaly

Polycythemia

Hypokalemia

Primary renal glycosuria

Primary polydipsia

Diabetes insipidus (central)

Diabetes insipidus (nephrogenic)

Diagnostic Approach

History and Physical Examination

✓ Estimate water intake when possible; animals with diabetes insipidus and primary polydipsia drink the largest amounts of water.

✋ Differentiate polyuria from pollakiuria and incontinence.

✓ Evidence of another disease such as diabetes mellitus, hyperadrenocorticism, renal failure, etc., may be gained from the history.

✓ Recent medications administered, including topical and ocular treatments should be noted.

✓ Physical examination may reveal lymphadenopathy or anal sac mass (hypercalcemia), enlarged uterus (pyometra), endocrine alopecia (hyperadrenocorticism), palpable thyroid mass (hyperthyroidism), abnormal kidney size or shape (renal failure, pyelonephritis), hepatomegaly (diabetes mellitus, hyperadreno-corticism, hepatic failure), bradycardia (hypoadrenocorticism), cataracts (diabetes mellitus), dehydration, or other changes.

Routine Laboratory Tests

Urinalysis

☛ Hyposthenuria (specific gravity < 1.008), isosthenuria (specific gravity 1.008-1.012), or minimally concentrated urine (1.013-1.025) should be present if PU/PD exists.

✓ Persistent hyposthenuria is most consistent with central or nephrogenic diabetes insipidus, primary polydipsia, and hypera-drenocorticism.

✓ Hyposthenuria generally eliminates renal failure as a potential cause.

✓ Pyuria or bacteriuria could be indicative of pyelonephritis, but there is a high incidence of urinary tract infection in animals with diabetes mellitus, hyperadrenocorticism or poorly concen-trated urine.

✓ Urine culture should be considered in any animal with isosthenuria regardless of urine sediment results as the dilute urine and underlying disease process may reduce white blood cell and/or bacteria numbers.

✓ Glycosuria is suggestive of diabetes mellitus or renal tubular dysfunction (primary renal glycosuria, Fanconi syndrome).

Complete Blood Count

✓ Infections such as pyelonephritis and pyometra may cause leukocytosis.

✓ Anemia may be present in animals with chronic renal failure, hypoadrenocorticism, or neoplasia.

Serum Biochemistries

✓ Azotemia is present in renal failure, but can also occur without renal failure in dogs with hypercalcemia. Prerenal azotemia can occur in hypoadrenocorticism and in animals with severe PU/PD and dehydration.

✓ Decreased BUN may be present in dogs or cats with hepatic insufficiency or central diabetes insipidus.

✓ Elevated liver enzymes can occur in hyperadrenocorticism (primarily alkaline phosphatase), diabetes mellitus, and hepatic disease and associated hepatic insufficiency.

✓ Significant hyperglycemia is consistent with diabetes mellitus when glycosuria is present; stress and hyperadrenocorticism should be ruled out as potential causes.

✓ Hypercalcemia may be due to hypercalcemia of malignancy, hypoadrenocorticism, renal failure, primary hyperparathyroidism or other disorders.

✓ Hypercholesterolemia in patients with PU/PD can be caused by hyperadrenocorticism and diabetes mellitus.

✓ Hypokalemia can directly cause PU/PD and has many causes including hyperaldosteronism, diabetes mellitus, gastrointestinal losses, and renal insufficiency.

✓ Hyperkalemia is found associated with PU/PD in hypoadrenocorticism and polyuric acute or end-stage chronic renal failure.

✓ Hyponatremia may be present in animals that have PU/PD with hypoadrenocorticism, primary polydipsia, hepatic failure with associated ascites, and renal failure. Hyponatremia may impair renal concentrating ability regardless of the cause.

✓ Hypernatremia in animals with PU/PD occurs with dehydration due to inadequate water intake when the cause of PU/PD is decreased secretion or impaired action of antidiuretic hormone (ADH). Causes include central or nephrogenic diabetes insipidus, hyperadrenocorticism, hypercalcemia, hepatic failure, pyometra, pyelonephritis, and hypokalemia.

Serum T4

✔ Hyperthyroidism is confirmed by finding an elevated serum T4 concentration in an animal with appropriate clinical signs.

Further Diagnostics

✔ A diagnosis can be made or differential diagnoses substantially refined based on routine laboratory testing for most cases of PU/PD.

♥ When no abnormalities are found on routine CBC and serum chemistries, central or nephrogenic diabetes insipidus, primary polydipsia, renal insufficiency (prior to development of azotemia), hyperadrenocorticism, and chronic pyelonephritis should be considered as likely differential diagnoses.

✔ Diabetes insipidus and primary polydipsia are very rare diseases.

Adrenal Function Testing

🐾 Consider testing for hyperadrenocorticism even if classical signs of the disease are not present because it induces a combination of secondary central and nephrogenic diabetes insipidus that is difficult to differentiate from primary diabetes insipidus based on results of water deprivation test.

Renal Imaging Studies

✔ Ultrasound examination abnormalities of pyelonephritis include dilated renal pelvis and proximal ureter and altered renal parenchymal echogenicity.

✔ Excretory urography may show renal pelvic or proximal ureteral dilation, blunting or distortion of the renal pelvic diverticula, and decreased dye opacity in the kidney and renal pelvis in cases of pyelonephritis and may be a more accurate test than ultrasound.

✔ These abnormalities are not specific for pyelonephritis and may persist after resolution of pyelonephritis; renal pelvic dilation may be present in animals with a variety of polyuric disorders or those receiving fluid therapy.

Glomerular Filtration Rate

Overview

✔ Persistent isosthenuria may occur in an animal with renal insufficiency before renal failure and azotemia occur.

✔ Glomerular filtration rate will allow for diagnosis of this difficult problem prior to performing a water deprivation test that can be dangerous in a dog with renal insufficiency.

✓ Methods include endogenous and exogenous creatinine clearance, clearance of inulin or iohexol, nuclear scintigraphy, and other techniques.

Protocol

✓ Endogenous creatinine clearance test:

1. Place indwelling urinary catheter (Foley) and empty bladder. Alternatively, repeated urethral catheterization can be performed.

2. Urine is collected for 8-24 hours, the volume recorded, and an aliquot is submitted to a laboratory for measurement of creatinine.

3. Obtain a blood sample at the end of the collection period for measurement of serum creatinine concentration.

4. Creatinine clearance = [urine volume (ml) x urine creatinine (mg/dl)]/[time (minutes) x serum creatinine (mg/dl) x body weight (kg)]

Interpretation

✓ Normal creatinine clearance is 2.0-4.5 ml/min/kg in dogs and 1.6-3.8 ml/min/kg in cats.

✓ Creatinine clearance must be considerably below normal to be compatible with renal insufficiency.

Limitations

✓ The finding of a reduced creatinine clearance does not ensure that it is the cause of the polyuria and polydipsia.

✓ The endogenous creatinine clearance is a relatively crude test, so a slight decrease may not be important.

Water Deprivation Test

Overview

♥ Should be performed only after all other appropriate testing has been undertaken.

💣※ Contraindicated if animal is dehydrated, or has azotemia or hypercalcemia.

✓ Protocol

Fast for 12 hours prior to and during the test.

1. Catheterize and empty urinary bladder.

2. Measure urine specific gravity.

3. Obtain body weight.

4. Obtain blood sample for measurement of BUN.

5. Withhold water.

6. Repeat 1-4 every 2 hours until one of the following criteria are met:

Urine specific gravity > 1.030
Weight loss of ≥ 5%
Azotemia
Clinical signs including depression, disorientation, vomiting
💣 It is essential to stop the water deprivation test if the animal loses >5% body weight, develops azotemia, or becomes ill; failure to do so may result in life-threatening dehydration and circulatory collapse.

7. After completion of the water deprivation test, administer desmopressin (DDAVP) 5 μg for cats and dogs < 15 kg and 10 μg for dogs > 15 kg IV or SQ; the intranasal preparation (100 μg/ml) can be used, but it is not sterile and should be passed through a bacteriostatic filter prior to use.

Empty bladder and record urine specific gravity 30, 60, 90, and 120 minutes after DDAVP administration.

8. At the end of the test, offer small amounts of water frequently, since consumption of large quantities could result in water intoxication and cerebral edema. Continue to monitor for signs of CNS depression or vomiting for 2 hours, after which water can be offered free choice.

Interpretation Prior to DDAVP Administration

✓ Concentration of urine specific gravity to > 1.030 is consistent with normal renal function and normal secretion and sensitivity to ADH which is consistent with primary polydipsia.

✓ Urine specific gravity of 1.008-1.020 is consistent with renal insufficiency, partial diabetes insipidus (central or nephrogenic, primary or secondary), and renal medullary washout with normal renal function.

✓ Urine specific gravity < 1.008 is consistent with complete central or nephrogenic diabetes insipidus or severe renal medullary washout, although some dogs with CDI have a urine specific gravity of up to 1.018.

Interpretation After DDAVP Administration

✓ Urine specific gravity should increase in dogs with CDI or primary polydipsia, but the increase may only be up to 1.018 in some cases.

✓ Renal medullary washout may prevent concentration of urine.

9

✔ Little or no increase in urine specific gravity will occur in nephrogenic diabetes insipidus.

Limitations

♥ It is essential to rule out all diseases except primary central or nephrogenic diabetes insipidus and primary polydipsia since many diseases (pyelonephritis, hypercalcemia, hypokalemia, pyometra, hyperadrenocorticism, hepatic failure, hyperthyroidism) that cause PU/PD affect ADH action on the renal collecting ducts causing a form of partial nephrogenic diabetes insipdus.

✔ Renal medullary washout will impair renal concentrating ability and may cause a misdiagnosis of diabetes insipidus.

♥ A 3-day, gradual water restriction to re-establish the renal medullary concentration gradient before complete water deprivation may be useful if the initial water deprivation test is nondiagnostic.

✔ Many animals require more than 10-12 hours to reach the end-point of the study, making it difficult to perform this test during regular clinic hours.

✔ If an animal fails to reach the end-point during this time, either the animal is transferred to an emergency facility overnight to continue the test, or the test is terminated and the animal can, several days later, have water withdrawn at midnight the night before admission for another water deprivation test.

✔ Measurement of plasma ADH may be necessary in some cases to make a diagnosis; ADH assay is available at many human laboratories.

ADH (DDAVP) Trial

Overview

✔ A simple test to differentiate central diabetes insipidus from nephrogenic diabetes insipidus is administration of DDAVP.

Protocol

✔ Have owners monitor water intake and obtain a urine sample for measurement of specific gravity for 2-3 days prior to testing.

✔ Administer 1-4 drops of DDAVP twice per day into the conjunctival sac for 5-7 days.

✔ Monitor water intake daily during this period.

✔ Evaluate urine specific gravity after 5-7 days.

Interpretation

✓ A positive response, diagnostic of central diabetes insipidus is a decrease in water intake by more than 50% and concentration of urine within 5-7 days of treatment.

✓ Partial nephrogenic diabetes insipidus may give a similar, but possibly less dramatic response.

✓ Complete nephrogenic diabetes insipidus should result in no response to DDAVP.

✓ Dogs with primary polydipsia may have some decrease in urine output and water consumption, but it is likely that excessive water consumption will persist.

Limitations

✓ All other possible causes of PU/PD should be eliminated prior to this test being performed for it to be valid.

✓ Any disorder causing secondary partial nephrogenic diabetes insipidus (including hyperadrenocorticism) could have a positive response similar to that of central diabetes insipidus.

✓ Renal medullary washout may prevent highly concentrated urine from being formed even in animals with central diabetes insipidus, but there should still be a substantial decrease in water consumption.

💣 Water intoxication is possible if excessive water consumption continues despite concentration of urine in dogs with primary polydipsia.

Diabetes Insipidus

Overview

✓ Central diabetes insipidus (CDI) is a rare disorder that occurs when there is deficient production of ADH.

✓ The cause of CDI is unknown in most cases, but includes neoplasia, congenital deficiencies of ADH, and trauma.

✓ CDI is commonly associated with pituitary or other intracranial neoplasia in older dogs.

✓ A partial deficiency of ADH (partial CDI) can result in the retention of some ability to concentrate urine.

Common Clinical Signs
✓ Polyuria and polydipsia are present in all cases.

✓ Urinary incontinence is a common complaint.

✓ Physical examination is typically normal unless neurologic signs caused by CNS neoplasia or trauma are present.

Routine Laboratory Tests
♥ Hyposthenuria is present in most cases.

✓ Urine specific gravity should not exceed 1.012, but dogs with a partial deficiency of ADH may be able to concentrate their urine slightly.

✓ Urinary tract infection is common because of dilute urine and urinary incontinence.

✓ Hypernatremia or hyponatremia may be present.

✓ Occasional abnormalities include decreased BUN, elevated alkaline phosphatase.

Specific Tests for Diagnosis
Water Deprivation Test
Interpretation
✓ Animals with complete diabetes insipidus should have minimal increase in urine specific gravity (≤ 1.012) after 5% dehydration.

✓ Partial diabetes insipidus may result in some ability to concentrate urine, but the specific gravity rarely exceeds 1.018.

✓ ADH or DDAVP administration after 5% dehydration on the water deprivation test typically results in an increase in urine specific gravity, but the increase may be mild. The usual range is 1.018 to 1.030.

✓ If plasma ADH is measured, it should be low prior to initiation of water deprivation and should not increase substantially after dehydration.

ADH (DDAVP) Trial
Interpretation
✓ A decrease in water consumption by greater than 50% is seen with complete CDI.

Treatment Recommendations

Objectives

✓ Resolve the PU/PD by increasing urine concentration.

Treatment

✓ DDAVP is administered into the conjunctival sac. The intranasal preparation is administered at 1-4 drops once per day.

✓ The frequency of administration can be increased if moderate to severe PU/PD occurs prior to administration of the next dose.

✓ The dose is adjusted weekly during initial treatment to find the dose that controls the severe PU/PD and secondarily to result in concentrated urine.

✓ An oral form of DDAVP is available but little is known about its use in dogs and cats; an initial dose of 0.1 mg PO BID-TID can be given, with an increase in dose by 0.05 mg weekly if an inadequate response is noted.

Monitoring Treatment

✓ Water consumption can be estimated by the owner and treatment tailored to maintain near normal water consumption or moderately concentrated urine based on measurements of urine specific gravity.

Complications of Treatment

✓ The only significant side effect is hyponatremia because of water intoxication from excessive water consumption after the urine becomes concentrated.

✓ Neurologic signs including vomiting, salivation, depression, ataxia, and seizures may occur with severe hyponatremia.

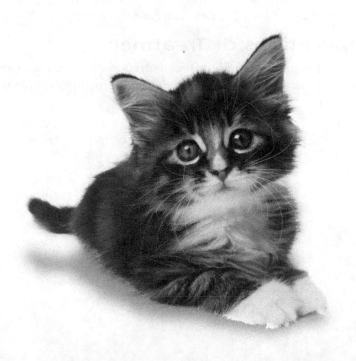

Section 2
Disorders of Growth Hormone

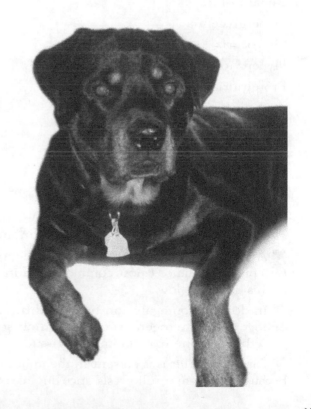

Acromegaly

♥ **Problems**

Polyuria, polydipsia

Polyphagia

Diabetes mellitus

Insulin resistance

Organomegaly (liver, kidneys, heart)

Increased body weight

Prognathia

Enlarged head

Widened interdental spaces

Enlarged tongue

Stridor

Heart murmur, cardiomyopathy

Lameness due to degenerative arthropathy

Renal failure

Hyperglycemia

Glycosuria

Hypercholesterolemia

Proteinuria

Azotemia

Hyperphosphatemia

Elevated liver enzymes

Erythrocytosis

Overview

✓ Acromegaly (hypersomatotropism) is the syndrome caused by chronic hypersecretion of growth hormone in an adult animal.

♥ Acromegaly can result from excessive growth hormone secretion by a pituitary tumor (most common form in the cat). The incidence of this disease is low.

♥ In dogs, acromegaly can be caused by excessive progestogens of endogenous or exogenous origin, which stimulate secretion of growth hormone from mammary tissue.

♥ Diabetes mellitus is present in the majority of affected animals because of severe insulin resistance due to excessive growth hormone.

♥ Complications of chronic acromegaly can be severe and include renal failure, heart failure secondary to hypertrophic cardiomyopathy, CNS signs due to a large pituitary tumor, and degenerative arthropathy.

Clinical Signs

Cats

♥ Clinical signs of diabetes mellitus, including polydipsia, polyuria, and polyphagia, are most common.

🖐 Weight gain rather than the weight loss expected in a poorly controlled diabetic may occur in about 50% of cases. This can also occur with chronic insulin overdose.

✓ Enlarged head, abdomen, and tongue, and prognathia may be observed (Figure 2-1).

✓ Hepatomegaly and renomegaly may be palpable.

✓ Heart murmur is common, and congestive heart failure can occur as the disease advances.

✓ Lameness and joint pain due to degenerative arthropathy are common in prolonged acromegaly.

✓ Upper respiratory stridor due to increased pharyngeal soft tissue can occur.

✓ Obtundation, stupor, seizures, circling, behavioral changes, and other neurologic abnormalities may occur due to an enlarging pituitary neoplasm.

✓ Some cats with acromegaly have insulin-resistant diabetes mellitus as the only clinical finding.

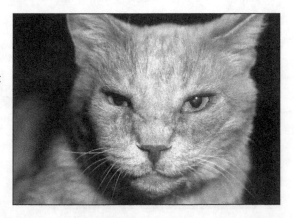

Figure 2-1 Neutered male cat with acromegaly and insulin resistant diabetes mellitus. Note the broad head, similar to that of an intact male.

Dogs

♥ Most dogs with acromegaly have a history of treatment with a progestogen or are an intact female that often have the onset of clinical signs concurrent with diestrous.

✓ Inspiratory stridor due to increased pharyngeal soft tissue is common.

✓ Diabetes mellitus may be present.

✓ Soft tissue and bone proliferation results in thickened skin and excessive skin folds around the head and neck, an enlarged head and abdomen, thickened limbs, and increased interdental spaces (Figures 2-2 and 2-3).

✓ Diabetes mellitus may be present.

✓ Mammary nodules (hyperplasia or neoplasia), vaginal discharge, and pyometra may be other consequences of progestogen administration.

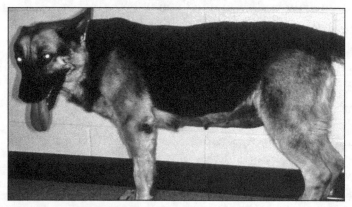

Figure 2-2 Intact female dog with progesterone-induced acromegaly and diabetes mellitus during diestrus. Note the "stocky" appearance due to thickened skin folds. The clinical signs and diabetes mellitus resolved following ovariohysterectomy.

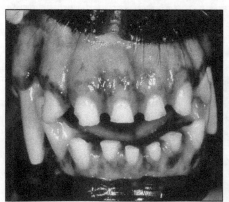

Figure 2-3 Widened interdental spaces in the same dog as in Figure 2-2.

Routine Laboratory Tests

✓ Erythrocytosis and mild leukocytosis are sometimes present.

✓ Hyperglycemia is present in almost all cats and many dogs.

✓ Glycosuria due to hyperglycemia associated with diabetes mellitus.

✓ Proteinuria of renal origin is common in cats secondary to glomerular injury possibly because of the diabetes mellitus and hypersomatotropism.

✓ Azotemia and renal failure are common in advanced cases of acromegaly in cats.

✓ Hyperproteinemia, hypercholesterolemia, elevated liver enzymes, and hyperphosphatemia are also found.

Diagnostic Imaging

✓ Changes are more common and more severe in cats.

✓ Radiographs of the head may reveal increased pharyngeal soft tissue and hyperostosis and periosteal proliferation of the skull.

✓ Degenerative arthropathy causes periarticular soft tissue swelling and periosteal proliferation with formation of osteophytes.

✓ Hepatomegaly and renomegaly are noted on abdominal radiographs and ultrasound.

✓ Cardiomegaly may be marked on thoracic radiographs.

✓ Echocardiography reveals ventricular hypertrophy with or without left atrial dilation.

♥ In cats, CT or MRI of the pituitary will reveal a mass consistent with a pituitary tumor in most cases (Figure 2-4).

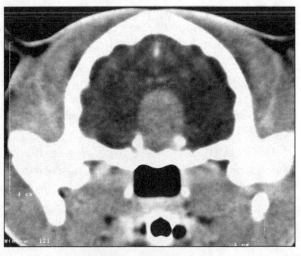

Figure 2-4 Contrast enhanced pituitary mass in a cat with acromegaly.

Specific Tests for Diagnosis

✓ Serum growth hormone concentration is elevated in dogs and cats with acromegaly.

♥ Assays for canine and feline growth hormone are not readily available.

♥ Insulin-like growth factor-1 (IGF-1, somatomedin C) is a protein that is produced in response to growth hormone. Elevated serum IGF-1 concentration is present in most animals with acromegaly.

✋ IGF-1 may be increased as a result of prolonged insulin administration. Therefore, IGF-1 may be elevated in diabetic cats that have been administered exogenous insulin for over 1 year, in the absence of growth hormone excess.

♥ Clinical signs consistent with acromegaly in a cat with insulin resistant diabetes mellitus of unknown cause is highly suggestive of acromegaly. Hyperadrenocorticism must be ruled out in these cases.

✓ Finding a mass in the pituitary gland on CT or MRI is suggestive of acromegaly if the clinical signs are appropriate and hyperadreno-corticism is not present.

Treatment Recommendations

♥ If acromegaly in a dog is due to progestogen excess, cessation of progestin administration or ovariohysterectomy should be curative.

✓ If present, diabetes mellitus may resolve if the acromegaly has not been long-standing.

♥ It is difficult to reduce the excess growth hormone secretion in cases of pituitary tumors, so much of the treatment of acromegaly is directed managing the complications of the disease, including diabetes mellitus, renal failure, cardiac disease and failure, and arthropathy.

✓ Specific treatment of the pituitary tumor is best accomplished by external-beam irradiation. Some cats will respond well with resolution of signs of acromegaly and diabetes mellitus. Recurrence of acromegaly is possible.

✓ Medical therapy to reduce growth hormone secretion using the somatostatin analog, octreotide, has not been successful. Few cases have been reported where octeotide has been used.

✓ A growth hormone receptor antagonist, pegvisomant, has been used successfully in humans, but its use has not been reported in animals with acromegaly.

✓ L-deprenyl (selegiline), through its action to increase dopamine, has been successful in treatment of some humans with acromegaly, although most do not respond. While L-deprenyl has not been effective in the only cat treated for acromegaly, it may be a practical treatment to attempt.

✓ Transphenoidal hypophysectomy has been used successfully for management of pituitary-dependent hyperadrenocorticism in cats and may be useful in cats with acromegaly. Access to surgeons with adequate skill and experience with this technique is limited.

Prognosis

✓ Progestogen-induced acromegaly resolves after eliminating the source of progestin, but diabetes mellitus sometimes persists.

✓ When the hypersomatotropism is not controlled in cats with pituitary tumors, the median survival is about 21 months. Renal failure, heart failure, and CNS signs are the most common causes of death or euthanasia.

Congenital Growth Hormone Deficiency (Pituitary Dwarfism)

♥ **Problems**

Stunted growth

Proportionate dwarfism

Retained puppy (lanugo) coat

Alopecia

Overview

✓ Congenital deficiency of growth hormone is a rare disease.

✓ German Shepherds account for most cases, but it can occur in other breeds of dog and in cats.

✓ A pituitary cyst is usually present, but its relationship to growth hormone deficiency appears to be coincidental.

Clinical Signs

♥ Animals are small but normally proportioned, unlike dogs with congenital hypothyroidism and most other causes of dwarfism.

✓ Dwarfism is noted within the first 3-5 months of life.

✓ The hair coat is soft and wooly due to retention of lanugo hairs and failure of primary hairs to grow.

✓ Thin skin with hyperpigmentation.

✓ As dogs age, they become dull and lethargic, perhaps secondary to development of hypothyroidism or hypoadrenocorticism.

Routine Laboratory Testing

✓ No specific abnormalities are found, but azotemia, hypoalbuminemia, and anemia may develop due to deficiency of growth hormone or other hormones.

Diagnostic Imaging

✓ Delayed closure of growth plates of long bones is the only common radiologic abnormality. This helps differentiate pituitary dwarfism from congenital hypothyroidism where epiphyseal growth is reduced and bones, including the vertebral bodies, are shortened.

✓ Pituitary imaging by MRI or CT may reveal a pituitary cyst, but cysts can also occur in normal dogs.

Specific Tests for Diagnosis

✓ A definitive diagnosis requires measurement of growth hormone during a stimulation test.

Measure growth hormone 0, 15, and 30 minutes after IV administration of xylazine (0.1 mg/kg), clonidine (10 µg/kg), or growth hormone releasing hormone (1 µg/kg). Clonidine is the preferred secretagogue.

Growth hormone concentrations should be low with minimal response to stimulation in pituitary dwarfism.

♥ Valid assays for canine growth hormone are very limited and a tentative diagnosis may be made in the absence of growth hormone measurement.

✓ Measurement of serum IGF-1 may be useful, but normal concentrations in growing dogs vary depending on breed. Large dogs have higher normal concentrations than small dogs.

♥ Thyroid and adrenal function should also be assessed as TSH and ACTH secretion can be decreased in pituitary dwarfism.

🖐 Secondary hypothyroidism and hypoadrenocorticism may not develop for many months after diagnosis of pituitary dwarfism.

Treatment Recommendations

✓ Human or bovine growth hormone can be administered (0.1 IU/kg 3 times per week) for 4-6 weeks.

✓ Response to treatment is usually fair to poor. Dogs may develop antibodies to the administered growth hormone that will make long-term treatment unsuccessful.

💣※ Diabetes mellitus may develop if treatment is given over a prolonged period.

♥ Administration of a progestogen (medroxyprogesterone acetate 2.5-5 mg/kg q 3 weeks) will stimulate endogenous growth hormone and IGF-1 production, and has been used successfully in treating growth hormone deficiency. Side effects include recurrent pyoderma, pruritus, cystic endometrial hyperplasia, and possibly mammary neoplasia.

Prognosis

✓ Guarded to poor, because of the ineffectiveness of long-term growth hormone administration and development of secondary hypothyroidism and hypoadrenocorticism.

♥ Long-term administration of a progestogen with concurrent management of other endocrinopathies probably provides the best opportunity for a good quality of life.

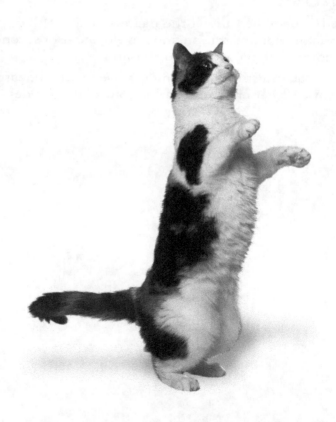

Section 3
Hypothyroidism

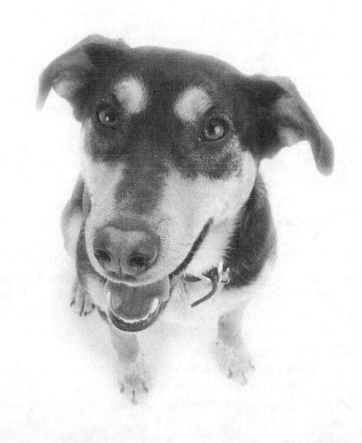

♥ **Problems**

Alopecia

Pyoderma

Seborrhea

Otitis externa

Weakness

Muscle atrophy

Hyporeflexia

Ataxia

Head tilt

Nystagmus

Facial nerve paralysis

Obesity

Hypercholesterolemia

Hyponatremia

Anemia

Bradycardia

Muffled heart sounds

Weak pulse

Hypothermia

Galactorrhea

Infertility

Macroglossia

Disproportionate dwarfism

Overview

✓ Hypothyroidism is the most common endocrine disorder in the dog.

✓ The vast majority of cases are primary hypothyroidism caused by either autoimmune thyroiditis or idiopathic thyroid gland atrophy.

✓ Spontaneous hypothyroidism is rare in the cat, with most cases being iatrogenic following treatment of hyperthyroidism.

✓ Canine hypothyroidism typically occurs in middle-aged, purebred dogs, with Golden Retrievers and Doberman Pinschers having the highest incidence of disease.

✓ Middle age and older dogs are most commonly affected.

Common Clinical Signs

General

♥ Obesity (usually mild) due to decreased metabolic rate is present in about 50% of hypothyroid dogs.

✓ Weakness and exercise intolerance are present in about 20%.

Dermatologic

♥ Dry, scaly skin and hair coat, alopecia, seborrhea, and hyperpigmentation are present to some degree in over 80% of hypothyroid dogs.

✓ The alopecia generally is first noted over areas of friction including the tail, neck, and ventral thorax (Figures 3-1 and 3-2). With prolonged hypothyroidism, most breeds will develop bilaterally symmetrical truncal alopecia (Figure 3-3).

✓ Pyoderma, otitis externa, change in hair color, and myxedema (non-pitting edema due to accumulation of mucopolysaccharides in the dermis) occur less frequently.

✓ Pruritus is absent unless concurrent bacterial or yeast infection is present.

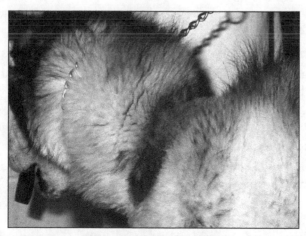

Figure 3-1 Alopecia of the neck and hyperpigmentation where a collar was located in a 5 year-old Alaskan Malamute with hypothyroidism.

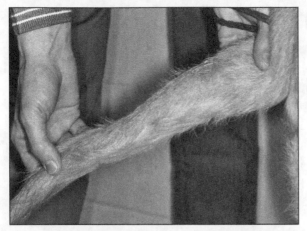

Figure 3-2 Alopecia of tail ("rat tail") in a 7-year-old Labrador Retriever with severe hypothyroidism.

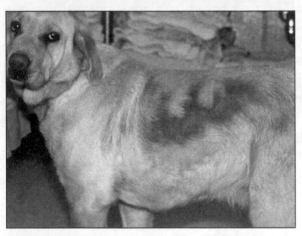

Figure 3-3 Bilaterally symmetrical truncal alopecia and hyperpigmentation in a hypothyroid dog.

Neurologic

✓ Peripheral neuropathy is diagnosed in 5-10% of hypothyroid dogs.

✓ Generalized polyneuropathy is manifested as generalized weakness, ataxia, and hyporeflexia.

✓ Localized neuropathies occur with a similar frequency to the generalized form, with vestibular and facial nerve paralysis occurring most commonly.

✓ Megaesophagus has been diagnosed in hypothyroid dogs, but the relationship between these disorders is unclear.

✓ Central nervous system signs (cerebellar or central vestibular), including head tilt, paresis, circling, strabismus, nystagmus, facial nerve paralysis, and trigeminal nerve dysfunction have been noted in a small number of hypothyroid dogs.

Cardiovascular

✓ Clinical signs of cardiac dysfunction are uncommon in hypothyroid dogs, but most probably have some degree of decreased myocardial function.

✓ Bradycardia is occasionally present (10-25%), and weak pulses or muffled heart sounds are also found.

✓ Electrocardiographic abnormalities including diminished R-wave amplitude (40-60%) and prolonged PR interval (10-20%) are common.

✓ Decreased myocardial contractility is sometimes present on echocardiography, but hypothyroidism only rarely causes reversible dilated cardiomyopathy and heart failure in the dog.

Uncommon Clinical Signs

Reproduction

✓ Female dogs with hypothyroidism may have reproductive abnormalities including infertility, prolonged anestrus, and short estrus.

🖑 Fertility in male dogs is not significantly affected by prolonged hypothyroidism.

✓ Galactorrhea can occur in intact females weeks to months beyond the normal period of diestrus, appearing to be prolonged pseudopregnancy.

Myxedema Stupor or Coma

✓ A very rare and life-threatening manifestation of hypothyroidism is myxedema coma.

♥ Hypothermia without shivering, severe depression progressing to coma, bradycardia, hypotension, non-pitting edema, and anorexia may be present.

✓ Hyponatremia, lipemia, hypercholesterolemia, hypoglycemia, and hypercapnea may be found on laboratory testing.

Ocular Disorders

✓ A variety of ocular disorders attributed to hypothyroidism, including corneal lipid dystrophy, corneal ulcers, anterior uveitis, retinal disease, and keratoconjunctivitis sicca, are rarely, if ever, truly caused by hypothyroidism.

Congenital Hypothyroidism

✓ Disproportionate dwarfism, large, broad head, short limbs, macroglossia, delayed dental eruption, coarse hair coat, abdominal distension, constipation, lethargy, obtundation, and ataxia are signs of congenital hypothyroidism.

✓ Puppies may be difficult to train because of impaired development of the central nervous system.

Feline Hypothyroidism

✓ Spontaneous hypothyroidism is very rare in the cat, with most cases being iatrogenic secondary to treatment of hyperthyroidism by surgical thyroidectomy or radioiodine.

✓ Clinical signs are similar to those of canine hypothyroidism, including seborrhea, hair coat abnormalities, obesity, lethargy, bradycardia, and hypothermia.

Routine Laboratory Tests

✓ Mild, nonregenerative anemia is present in approximately 25% of hypothyroid dogs.

♥ Hypercholesterolemia is the most consistent biochemical abnormality, occurring in 75% of cases.

✓ Hyponatremia, elevated alkaline phosphatase, alanine aminotransferase, and creatine kinase activities occur less frequently.

Diagnostic Imaging

✓ Diagnostic imaging is of little use in the evaluation of dogs and cats with adult-onset hypothyroidism.

✓ Radiographic abnormalities in congenital hypothyroidism include epiphyseal dysgenesis and poor ephiphyseal ossification resulting in shortened vertebrae, poorly calcified vertebrae and long bones, and delayed and retarded growth of the epiphyses of long bones.

Specific Tests for Diagnosis

Primary Tests

⚷ The pattern of thyroid function tests most diagnostic of primary hypothyroidism is decreased serum T4 and fT4 and elevated serum TSH concentrations.

♥ Patient selection is important, and dogs with significant nonthyroidal illness and those receiving drugs known to affect thyroid function tests should be tested after resolution of the illness or discontinuation of the drug if possible.

Serum Total Thyroxine (T4) Concentration

Overview

♥ Serum T4 is a sensitive, but not specific test for the diagnosis of canine hypothyroidism.

✓ It should be included in any battery of tests used to evaluate thyroid function.

♥ Serum T4 is the primary test used for monitoring thyroid hormone replacement therapy.

Interpretation

♥ Serum T4 concentration is below the reference range in about 90% of hypothyroid dogs.

♥ It is also below normal in 20-25% of euthyroid dogs with some clinical signs of hypothyroidism.

⚷ A serum T4 concentration below normal in a dog with classical clinical signs of hypothyroidism and no overt concurrent illness is sufficient for a tentative diagnosis of hypothyroidism and warrants a clinical trial of thyroid hormone supplementation.

Limitations

✓ Nonthyroidal illness and certain drugs (sulfonamides, phenobarbital, glucocorticoids) will lower serum T4 concentrations.

✍ Dogs with moderate to severe illness should have thyroid function testing delayed until resolution of the nonthyroidal illness if possible.

✓ Autoantibodies to T4, which occur in up to 10% of hypothyroid dogs, will cause an elevation of measured T4 by interfering with the immunoassay. The increase may be mild (could increase the T4 into the normal range in a hypothyroid dog) or may be marked (serum T4 greatly elevated above the reference range mimicking hyperthyroidism).

Serum Free Thyroxine (fT4) Concentration by Equilibrium Dialysis

Overview

✓ Serum fT4 is a sensitive and relatively specific test for diagnosis of hypothyroidism when the assay is performed using the equilibrium dialysis technique.

🖐 If the equilibrium dialysis technique is not used, measurement of fT4 is of no advantage over that of total T4.

✓ Free T4 less affected by nonthyroidal factors than serum total T4.

Interpretation

♥ Serum fT4 has a similar sensitivity to total T4, being decreased in 90-98% of hypothyroid dogs.

✓ Serum fT4 is more specific than other thyroid function tests because it is less prone to the effects of nonthyroidal illness and is not affected by T4 autoantibodies and some drugs that affect total T4.

Limitations

✓ Drugs, including sulfonamides, glucocorticoids, and phenobarbital as well as severe illness and hyperadrenocorticism may decrease fT4 concentrations.

Serum Thyroid Stimulating Hormone (TSH) Concentration

Overview

✓ Secretion of TSH is controlled by the negative feedback of T4 and T3 on the pituitary gland (Figure 3-4). As thyroid hormones decrease in primary thyroid disease, TSH secretion increases. This results in normalization of thyroid hormone concentrations in the presence of elevated plasma TSH. With progressive destruction of the thyroid gland, T4 secretion eventually becomes inadequate despite elevated TSH concentrations. Thus, elevated TSH should be a hallmark of primary hypothyroidism in the dog as it is in man.

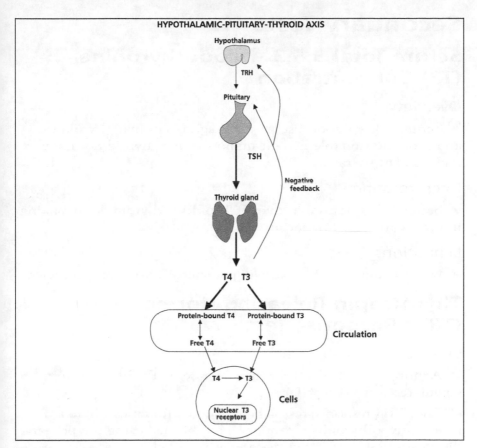

Figure 3-4 Hypothalamic-pituitary-thyroid axis.

Interpretation

♥ Serum TSH concentration is elevated in 65-75% of dogs with hypothyroidism.

✓ Serum TSH is elevated in 8-15% of euthyroid dogs with nonthyroidal illness and clinical signs compatible with hypothyroidism.

☞ Elevated serum TSH concentration in a dog with serum T4 and/or fT4 below the reference range is diagnostic of hypothyroidism in the absence of substantial nonthyroidal illness.

Limitations

♥ Serum TSH concentration is an insensitive test for hypothyroidism. A normal serum TSH concentration does not exclude a diagnosis of hypothyroidism.

✓ Serum TSH can be elevated in dogs with nonthyroidal illness that could lead to a misdiagnosis of hypothyroidism.

Secondary Tests

Serum Total 3,5,3'-triiodothyronine (T3) Concentration

Overview

♥ Serum T3 is a poor test for the diagnosis of hypothyroidism and is of questionable benefit in monitoring thyroid hormone replacement therapy.

Interpretation

✓ Serum T3 is normal in over 50% of hypothyroid dogs, making it a test with very low sensitivity.

Limitations

✓ Not recommended because of poor sensitivity and specificity.

Thyrotropin Releasing Hormone (TRH) Response Test

Overview

✓ Administration of TRH causes release of TSH that in turn stimulates secretion of T4.

✓ The TRH response test is best reserved for cases where a diagnosis of hypothyroidism cannot be established using the primary diagnostic tests and other diseases are unlikely.

Protocol

✓ Obtain a blood sample for measurement of serum T4 before and 4 hours after IV administration of 200 micrograms of TRH.

Interpretation

✓ A post-TRH serum T4 concentration greater than 25 nmol/L is considered normal.

Limitations

✓ Some normal dogs do not have an increase in T4 in response to TRH, so a diagnosis of hypothyroidism cannot really be confirmed using this test.

✓ The TRH response test is best used to rule out a diagnosis of hypothyroidism in a dog with a normal response.

✓ Depression, salivation, vomiting, defecation, and urination can occur transiently after TRH administration.

TSH Response Test

Overview

✓ Administration of TSH causes secretion of thyroid hormones. The TSH response test is considered the gold standard for diagnosis of hypothyroidism in the dog and cat.

✓ Rarely necessary for diagnosis of hypothyroidism.

Protocol

✓ Obtain a blood sample for measurement of serum T4 before and 6 hours after IV administration of 0.1 unit/kg up to a maximum 5 units of bovine TSH or 50 µg human recombinant TSH.

Interpretation

✓ A serum T4 concentration > 30 nmol/L is considered normal.

✓ Most hypothyroid dogs have little if any increase in T4 following administration and typically have pre and post-TSH T4 concentrations < 20 nmol/L.

Limitations

✓ Pharmaceutical grade bovine TSH is no longer available and human recombinant TSH is very costly.

Autoantibodies to T4 and T3

Overview

✓ Thyroid hormone autoantibodies occur occasionally in dogs with lymphocytic thyroiditis.

✓ The importance of thyroid hormone autoantibodies lies in their ability to interfere with measurement of serum T4 and/or T3, usually resulting in a marked elevation of T4 and T3 without causing hyperthyroidism.

✓ Free T4 by equilibrium dialysis must be used to accurately evaluate thyroid function in the presence of T4 autoantibodies.

✓ These autoantibodies also act as a marker of autoimmune thyroiditis.

Antithyroglobulin Antibodies

Overview

✓ This is not a test of thyroid function, but rather a serologic marker of autoimmune thyroiditis. It may be useful in identifying dogs with thyroiditis, but does not aid in the diagnosis of hypothyroidism.

Therapeutic Trial with Levothyroxine Treatment

Overview

✓ Administration of a therapeutic dose of levothyroxine without adequate thyroid function testing has been suggested as a diagnostic test for hypothyroidism, but is not recommended.

✓ Clinical signs should resolve if the dog is hypothyroid and there should be no response if it is not.

Protocol

✓ Obtain history and physical examination after treatment for 6-8 weeks of levothyroxine treatment (0.02 mg/kg q 12 h).

♥ If a positive response has occurred, treatment should be withdrawn and the dog re-examined in 4-6 weeks.

Interpretation

✓ Resolution of clinical signs during treatment and recurrence after withdrawing treatment is highly suggestive of hypothyroidism.

✓ Failure to respond to treatment or lack of recurrence of clinical signs after cessation of treatment eliminates hypothyroidism as a diagnosis.

Limitations

♥ Dogs suspected of hypothyroidism are often treated with other medications such as antibiotics for pyoderma, topical medications for dermatologic abnormalities, and other treatments that could account for the clinical response when used concurrent with levothyroxine.

✓ Levothyroxine does have supraphysiologic effects including increased hair growth and activity that could be mistaken for a therapeutic response and result in a misdiagnosis of hypothyroidism.

Treatment Recommendations

Objectives

✓ To resolve the metabolic abnormalities associated with hypothyroidism by approximating normal secretion of thyroid hormones.

Treatment

♥ Levothyroxine should be administered initially at 0.02 mg/kg twice per day.

✓ Because some dogs respond better to twice daily therapy, once per day treatment should only be considered after resolution of clinical signs.

🐾 Dogs with congestive heart failure, diabetes mellitus, hypoadrenocorticism, renal failure, and hepatic insufficiency should have treatment initiated with 25% of the normal replacement dose, and gradual increases in dose (increase by 25% every two weeks) based on clinical response and measurement of serum T4 concentration.

✓ Treatment with other preparations including desiccated thyroid, thyroglobulin, combinations of T4 and T3, and liothyronine (synthetic T3) is unnecessary and would be more likely to result in iatrogenic hyperthyroidism.

Monitoring Treatment

✓ Clinical response as indicated by increased activity and improved attitude is usually noted within 1 week of initiating treatment.

✓ Other signs take longer to resolve, with dermatologic abnormalities sometimes requiring several months to resolve.

♥ Post-pill therapeutic monitoring is recommended for all dogs undergoing treatment for hypothyroidism because of the variable pharmacokinetics of levothyroxine.

✓ Measurement of T4 can be done as soon as 2 weeks after initiating treatment, but evaluation at 6-8 weeks allows time for clinical signs to respond to treatment.

♥ The appropriate 4-hour post-pill T4 concentration should be near or slightly above the upper limit of the reference range (40-70 nmol/L).

♥ If measured, serum TSH concentration should be suppressed to within the normal range if treatment is adequate.

👋 If improvement in clinical signs has not occurred within 8 weeks of initiating treatment and post-pill serum T4 and TSH are in the therapeutic range, an alternative diagnosis should be considered.

Complications of Treatment

✔ Dogs are relatively resistant to developing clinical signs of hyperthyroidism when an overdose of levothyroxine is administered.

✔ Clinical signs of hyperthyroidism include polydipsia, polyuria, hyperactivity, panting, tachycardia, and weight loss.

✔ If these signs are noted, a serum sample for T4 should be obtained and the treatment should be stopped pending these results.

✔ If hyperthyroidism is induced by a standard dose of levothyroxine, the dog should be evaluated for conditions that might predispose it to hyperthyroidism, including renal failure or hepatic disease.

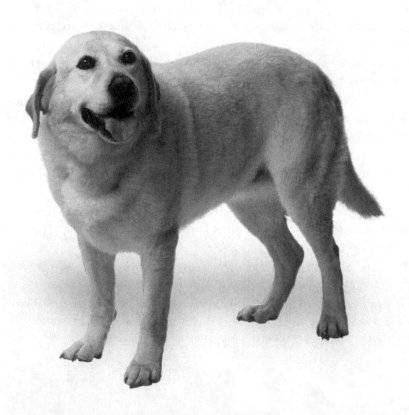

Section 4

Hyperthyroidism

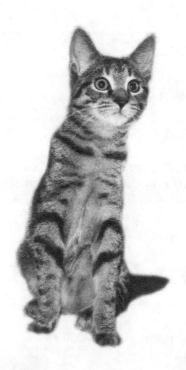

♥ Problems

Weight loss

Polyphagia

Poor hair coat

Polyuria/polydipsia

Vomiting

Hyperactivity

Diarrhea

Weakness

Panting

Anorexia

Decreased activity

Palpable thyroid gland enlargement

Thin body condition

Tachycardia

Heart murmur or gallop cardiac rhythm

Increased nail growth

Ventral flexion of the neck

Hypertension

Erythrocytosis

Elevated liver enzyme activity

Azotemia

Urine specific gravity <1.035

Overview

✓ Hyperthyroidism is a common disease of cats over 6 years of age. Feline hyperthyroidism is caused by adenomatous hyperplasia or adenoma of the thyroid gland; carcinomas are rare. The cause remains unknown.

✓ The disease is bilateral in 70% of cases.

Common Clinical Signs

General

✓ Weight loss is present in about 90% of cases, but many hyperthyroid cats are not thin.

✓ Polyphagia is present in about 50% of cases and is a response to increased metabolic rate and the subsequent increase in energy demands.

✓ Hyperactivity, apparent anxiousness, and excessive resistance to restraint during examination are present in over 1/3 of hyperthyroid cats.

✓ Decreased appetite or anorexia is occasionally reported.

♥ A ventral cervical mass (enlarged thyroid gland) is palpable in about 90% of cases (Figure 4-1).

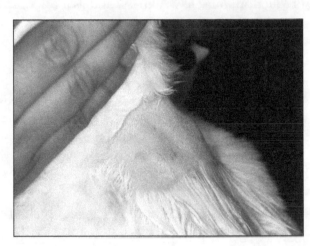

Figure 4-1 Large thyroid gland in the ventral cervical area of a cat with hyperthyroidism.

Renal
✓ Polyuria and polydipsia are present in about 50% of cases and are caused by either increased renal blood flow or concurrent renal failure.

Cardiovascular
✓ Heart murmur or gallop rhythm is ausculted in about 50% of cases.

✓ Congestive heart failure can occur secondary to hyperthyroidism, but is uncommon.

✓ Tachycardia is found in about 40% of cases; other cardiac arrhythmias occur infrequently.

🖑 Systemic arterial hypertension is common.

Dermatologic
✓ A poor, unkempt hair coat and alopecia are present in some hyperthyroid cats.

Gastrointestinal

✓ Vomiting occurs in about 40% of cases, possibly due to consuming large quantities of food rapidly.

✓ Diarrhea or increased fecal volume is present in about 20%.

Respiratory

✓ Panting or dyspnea is occasionally present in hyperthyroid cats and may be secondary to a variety of mechanisms including increased CO_2 production, muscle weakness, and as a response to stress.

Neurologic

✓ Generalized weakness can occur because of impaired muscle function.

✓ Cervical ventroflexion is occasionally present and may be due to myopathy, hypokalemia, or thiamine deficiency.

✓ Central nervous system signs can occur secondary to hypertension and subsequent brain hemorrhage.

Ocular

✓ Hypertensive retinopathy causing retinal hemorrhage, retinal detachment, and subretinal effusion may be present.

Canine Hyperthyroidism

✓ Hyperthyroidism is rare in the dog.

✓ Most thyroid tumors in dogs are malignant and only about 10% are functional.

✓ Clinical signs are similar to those found in cats with hyperthyroidism. A palpable, often large, thyroid mass is found in nearly all cases.

Routine Laboratory Tests

Complete Blood Count

✓ A slight increase in hematocrit and MCV is present in 40-50% of hyperthyroid cats.

✓ Leukocytosis, eosinopenia, and lymphopenia are sometimes present.

Serum Chemistries

♥ Elevated liver enzyme (ALT, AST, alkaline phosphatase) activity is commonly present; almost all hyperthyroid cats have an elevation of one or more of these enzymes.

✓ Mild hyperglycemia is present in 20%.

✓ BUN and creatinine are elevated in 30% of cats. Renal failure may be present in the majority of hyperthyroid cats with azotemia.

♥ Treatment of hyperthyroidism may result in worsening of azotemia and clinical signs of uremia in some cases.

Urinalysis

✓ Minimally concentrated urine with a specific gravity of 1.015-1.035 is common in cats with hyperthyroidism.

✓ Low urine specific gravity does not necessarily indicate impaired renal function since increased renal blood flow due to elevated cardiac output can impair renal concentrating ability.

Diagnostic Imaging

✓ In general, diagnostic imaging is not necessary for the diagnosis and management of the routine case of hyperthyroidism.

Thoracic Radiographs

✓ Indicated when dyspnea, tachypnea, or muffled heart and lung sounds are present.

✓ Cardiomegaly is commonly seen.

✓ Pleural effusion or pulmonary edema may be present in cats with congestive heart failure.

Echocardiography

✓ Indicated when there is congestive heart failure, cardiomegaly on radiographs, or a significant cardiac arrhythmia.

✓ Modest left ventricular hypertrophy and dilation with or without atrial enlargement is typical of the hyperthyroid heart.

✓ Some hyperthyroid cats have marked left ventricular hypertrophy that may be due to the hyperthyroidism or concurrent idiopathic hypertrophic cardiomyopathy.

✓ Myocardial failure and ventricular dilation is occasionally found in hyperthyroid cats; if associated with congestive heart failure it carries a poor prognosis.

Ultrasonography

✔ Abdominal ultrasound might be indicated in hyperthyroid cats with concurrent disease, but not in uncomplicated hyperthyroidism.

✔ Cervical ultrasound can identify enlarged thyroid glands, but is not necessary for diagnosis.

Ancillary Testing

Electrocardiography

✔ Indicated if an arrhythmia is suspected, if there is evidence of congestive heart failure, or if a hyperthyroid cat is to be anesthetized.

✔ Sinus tachycardia and left ventricular enlargement patterns are the most common findings.

✔ Atrial premature contractions and other supraventricular arrhythmias are more common than ventricular arrhythmias.

Arterial Blood Pressure

✔ Should be measured in all cases. Very important if signs of hypertension are present (neurologic signs, retinal effusion, hemorrhage or detachment).

Specific Tests for Diagnosis

Primary Tests

♥ Hyperthyroidism is usually readily diagnosed by documenting elevated serum total T4 concentration. Cats with a normal serum T4 and clinical signs of hyperthyroidism may have mild hyperthyroidism, hyperthyroidism with a concurrent nonthyroidal illness, or a disease other than hyperthyroidism. If the serum T4 is normal in a cat suspected of hyperthyroidism, a second serum T4 measurement 1- 4 weeks later, or a free T4 concentration should be measured. If these tests are inconclusive, a T3 suppression test or TRH stimulation test is indicated.

Serum Total Thyroxine (T4) Concentration

Overview
♥ Total T4 is a sensitive and specific test for diagnosis of hyperthyroidism and should be the first test performed.

Interpretation
♥ Serum total T4 is elevated in over 90% of hyperthyroid cats.

✔ An elevated T4 concentration is diagnostic of hyperthyroidism when the cat has appropriate clinical signs.

✔ If the total T4 is normal and hyperthyroidism is still suspected, serum T4 should be measured again in 1-4 weeks since T4 concentrations fluctuate in hyperthyroid cats. Alternatively, a serum free T4 concentration can be measured.

Limitations
✔ Cats with mild hyperthyroidism may have a normal total T4 (<10% of cases).

✔ Nonthyroidal illness can decrease total T4 into the normal range in hyperthyroid cats.

Serum Free Thyroxine by Equilibrium Dialysis (fT4) Concentration

Overview
✔ More sensitive than total T4 for diagnosis of hyperthyroidism: elevated in about 98% of hyperthyroid cats.

Less specific than total T4 (some false positive tests).

✔ Free T4 must be measured using the equilibrium dialysis assay to be useful. Other methods for estimating free T4 do not offer an advantage over measurement of total T4.

Interpretation
✔ Elevated free T4 in a cat without a concurrent nonthyroidal illness is diagnostic of hyperthyroidism.

♥ Free T4 may be invalid in cats with nonthyroidal illness, so fully evaluate the cat for other illnesses when using this test.

Limitations
♥ Elevated in 6-12% of cats with nonthyroidal illness, including some cats with mild illness. A misdiagnosis can be made in this situation, so always combine free T4 measurement with a serum total T4.

Secondary Tests

Serum Total 3,5,3'-triiodothyronine (T3) Concentration

Overview

♥ Serum T3 is frequently (>30%) normal in hyperthyroid cats, so it is a poor test for diagnosis of hyperthyroidism.

Interpretation

✓ Elevated T3 is diagnostic of hyperthyroidism.

✓ Normal T3 occurs commonly in hyperthyroid cats.

Limitations

✓ Insensitive test for the diagnosis of hyperthyroidism, therefore serum T3 is not recommended for routine use.

Thyrotropin Releasing Hormone (TRH) Stimulation Test

Overview

✓ Used when total T4 and fT4 are not diagnostic.

✓ As effective as the T3 suppression test in diagnosing hyperthyroidism in difficult cases.

Protocol

✓ Obtain blood sample for serum T4 concentration before and 4 hours after IV administration of 0.1 µg/kg TRH.

Interpretation

✓ Normal response is an increase in T4 on the 4 hour sample > 60% of the basal concentration.

✓ Hyperthyroidism is diagnosed when the increase in serum T4 concentration is < 50% of baseline.

Limitations

✓ Nonthyroidal illness can cause suppression of response in a normal cat, leading to a misdiagnosis of hyperthyroidism.

✓ Salivation, vomiting, defecation, and vocalization frequently occur transiently after administration of TRH.

✓ TRH is not readily available.

T3 Suppression Test

Overview
✓ Used when total T4 and fT4 are not diagnostic.

✓ As effective as the TRH stimulation test in diagnosing hyperthyroidism in difficult cases.

Protocol
✓ Prior to initiating test obtain blood sample for measurement of serum T4.

✓ Administer T3 at 25 µg PO q 8 hours for 7 doses.

✓ Obtain blood sample 2-4 hours after the final dose of T3 for measurement of serum T4 and T3 concentrations.

Interpretation
✓ Normal response is a decrease in T4 concentration to < 20 nmol/L.

✓ Hyperthyroidism is diagnosed when the serum T4 is > 20 nmol/L post-T3 administration.

✓ Serum T3 should be elevated on the post-treatment sample unless the T3 was not administered properly.

Limitations
♥ Requires administration of oral medication that may be difficult for owners to accomplish.

✓ Effects of nonthyroidal illness on this test are unknown.

Treatment Recommendations

Antithyroid Drug Treatment
♥ Methimazole is the drug of choice for medical management of hyperthyroidism.

✓ Carbimazole is metabolized to methimazole and is available in countries outside of North America.

✓ Methimazole inhibits synthesis of thyroid hormones, but does not affect secretion of preformed hormone.

🖐 Methimazole should be used prior to a more permanent treatment in order to assess the effects that resolution of hyperthyroidism has on renal function.

Objectives

✔ Reduce plasma thyroid hormone concentrations into the normal range.

Treatment

✔ Methimazole should initially be administered at 5 mg/day in a single dose or divided twice per day. Twice daily treatment may be more effective than a single daily dosage.

✔ Methimazole can be given orally or transdermally in a pleuronic lecithin organogel. Transdermal gel is usually compounded to a concentration of 50 mg/ml and applied to the inner pinna. The owner should wear a glove to prevent contact of the gel with skin. The pinna is cleaned with a moist cloth prior to application if necessary, and the gel is gently rubbed into the skin.

Monitoring Treatment

♥ Complete blood count should be evaluated every 2 weeks for the first 3 months of treatment to monitor for neutropenia, anemia, and thrombocytopenia.

♥ Renal function should be evaluated every 2 weeks until serum T4 concentration has decreased into the normal range.

✔ Measure serum T4 concentration every 2 weeks until it is within the low to mid-normal range. The dose of methimazole can be increased by 2.5 to 5 mg if serum T4 is not within the normal range after 4-6 weeks of treatment.

✔ Serum T4 concentration should be measured every 6-12 months after the disease is adequately controlled and the appropriate methimazole dose has been determined.

Complications of Treatment

♥ Anorexia, vomiting, and occasionally diarrhea are the most common side effects, particularly when methimazole is administered at high doses.

✔ If gastrointestinal side effects occur, discontinuation of treatment for 2-4 days followed by administration of a lower dose often allows treatment to proceed.

♦※ Severe hematologic side effects occur in about 4% of cases including agranulocytosis (granulocyte count < 500/µl), thrombocytopenia, and hemolytic anemia that can lead to sepsis or hemorrhage (Figure 4-2).

✔ Hepatopathy, and severe facial pruritus can also occur.

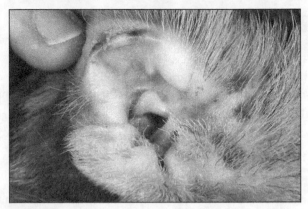

Figure 4-2 Petichiae on the pinna of a cat 3 weeks after initiating treatment with methimazole. The cat recovered after receiving a whole blood transfusion and discontinuing methimazole treatment.

✓ Side effects are reversible and generally resolve within 5 days of stopping methimazole.

💣 If hematologic, heptic, or cutaneous side effects occur, further methimazole administration is contraindicated.

♥ Renal failure may occur during methimazole treatment due to the decrease in renal blood flow and glomerular filtration rate that occur when the elevated cardiac output associated with hyperthyroidism resolves. The methimazole dosage should be adjusted to maintain serum T4 in the mid- to upper-normal range if azotamia develops.

Alternative Medical Treatments

Iopanoic Acid

✓ When methimazole is poorly tolerated, the most effective alternative with the fewest side effects is iopanoic acid.

✓ Iopanoic acid is an oral cholecystographic contrast agent that inhibits conversion of T4 to T3.

Objectives

✓ Reduce serum T3 concentration to within the normal range and eliminate signs of hyperthyroidism until a more definitive treatment can be undertaken.

✓ These agents have little effect on serum T4 concentrations.

Treatment

✓ Administer 50 mg twice per day.

Monitoring Treatment

✔ Measure serum T3 and assess clinical signs every 2 weeks until adequate response is seen.

✔ Adjust dose in 50 mg increments based on resolution of clinical signs and serum T3 concentration within the normal range.

✔ The response may be transient, with some cats suffering recurrence of hyperthyroidism despite continued treatment.

Complications of Treatment

✔ No side effects have been noted.

✔ A beta-adrenergic blocker (propranolol, atenolol) may be administered if tachycardia or other arrhythmia is present.

Radioactive Iodine

♥ Treatment of choice if available and affordable.

Objectives

✔ Destruction of hyperactive thyroid tissue by uptake of radioiodine; normal thyroid tissue should be spared in most cases.

Treatment

✔ Requires special facility for isolation and for disposal of radioactive waste.

✔ Cats should be otherwise relatively healthy to be good candidates for treatment.

✔ Methimazole treatment does not inhibit iodine uptake so its administration is generally recommended prior to radioiodine treatment. Withdrawal time prior to radioiodine administration is dependent on protocol of practice administering the ^{131}I.

✔ Administration of a single dose of 3-5 mCi ^{131}I by subcutaneous injection is effective.

✔ Treated cats are isolated for a variable period of time dependent on local regulations. Release to the owner occurs 3-21 days after radioiodine administration.

Monitoring Treatment

✔ Recheck serum T4 1-3 months after treatment; continued destruction of thyroid tissue can occur for many months after treatment in some cats.

✔ Most cats are euthyroid within 1-2 months of treatment.

Complications of Treatment

✓ Clinical signs of hypothyroidism occurs in about 2% of treated cats; about 10% have serum T4 below the normal range, but do not have clinical signs and do not require thyroid hormone supplementation.

♥ Decreased renal function may be noted as with any treatment of hyperthyroidism.

Percutaneous Ethanol Injection

Objectives

✓ Destruction of hyperplastic thyroid tissue by coagulation necrosis following injection.

Treatment

♥ Considerable expertise is required to safely perform this procedure.

✓ Ethanol (96%) is injected into the enlarged thyroid gland under ultrasound guidance until the entire thyroid gland is infiltrated with the cat under general anesthesia.

✋ Only one thyroid gland should be treated at a given time even if both thyroid glands are enlarged; the contralateral gland should be treated at a later date.

✓ Results with treatment of cats with unilateral involvement has been good, while hyperthyroidism has uniformly reoccurred in those with bilateral disease.

Complications of Treatment

☀ Laryngeal paralysis is a common complication, which may be permanent or transient; bilateral laryngeal paralysis may be fatal.

Surgical Thyroidectomy

✓ An effective, permanent treatment of hyperthyroidism.

Objectives

✓ Removal of all hyperplastic/neoplastic thyroid tissue with preservation of parathyroid gland function.

Treatment

♥ Bilateral thyroidectomy is recommended since 70% of cases have bilateral disease; both thyroids may be removed at the same time or the surgeries can be staged with 4-6 weeks between excisions of each thyroid lobe.

✓ Numerous surgical techniques have been described.

✓ Intracapsular procedures are more likely to preserve parathyroid function, but may leave hyperplastic tissue behind and lead to recurrence of hyperthyroidism.

✓ Extracapsular techniques may be more effective at removing affected thyroid tissue, but can lead to removal of external parathyroid glands or damage of the blood supply to the parathyroid gland.

♥ The parathyroid gland can be transplanted to an adjacent muscle belly if it is inadvertently removed.

✓ Levothyroxine supplementation (0.1 mg QD) is recommended for 2 months following bilateral thyroidectomy.

Monitoring Treatment

✋ Post-operative monitoring of serum calcium concentration after surgery is necessary when bilateral thyroidectomy is performed because of the danger of hypocalcemia.

✓ Although serum T4 concentration is often below normal after bilateral thyroidectomy, supplementation beyond the initial 2 months after surgery is rarely necessary.

Complications of Treatment

💣 Hypocalcemia is possible with bilateral thyroidectomy; daily measurement of serum calcium concentration is recommended for 3-5 days after surgery. See section 13 for management of hypocalcemia.

✓ Laryngeal paralysis and Horner's syndrome occur rarely due to intraoperative trauma.

✓ Permanent hypothyroidism is infrequent, but levothyroxine (0.1 mg PO QD) treatment should be instituted in cats with clinical signs of hypothyroidism and serum T4 concentration below normal. Dosage adjustments should be made based on clinical response and measurement of serum T4 during treatment. Clinical signs of hypothyroidism include lethargy, poor hair coat, seborrhea, and weight gain.

✓ Decreased renal function may be noted as with any treatment of hyperthyroidism.

✓ Levothyroxine supplementation sufficient to result in serum T4 concentration in the upper limit of the normal range should be considered if renal failure occurs.

Section 5

Hyperadrenocorticism

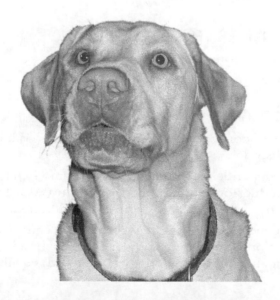

Canine Hyperadrenocorticism

♥ Problems

Polyuria

Polydipsia

Polyphagia

Weakness

Excessive panting

Obesity

Alopecia

Thin skin

Comedones

Calcinosis cutis

Recurrent pyoderma

Distended abdomen

Muscle wasting

Pseudomyotonia

Hepatomegaly

Hypertension

Isosthenuria or hyposthenuria

Proteinuria

Elevated alkaline phosphatase activity

Hypercholesterolemia

Erythrocytosis

Overview

✓ Hyperadrenocorticism (Cushing's syndrome) is a common endocrine disorder.

✓ Pituitary-dependent hyperadrenocorticism (PDH) is caused by excessive production of adrenocorticotropin (ACTH) by the pituitary gland, usually due to a pituitary adenoma.

✓ Adrenal-dependent hyperadrenocorticism is cause by excessive cortisol secretion by an adrenocortical adenoma or adenocarcinoma; benign and malignant adrenal tumors occur with equal frequency.

♥ PDH accounts for 80-85% of cases of hyperadrenocorticism, while adrenal tumors comprise 15-20%.

✓ Breeds most commonly affected include Poodles, Dachshunds, Boxers, and Boston Terriers, although hyperadrenocorticism can occur in any breed.

✓ Most dogs with hyperadrenocorticism are over 6 years of age.

Clinical Signs

♥ Polyuria and polydipsia are the most common clinical signs in dogs with hyperadrenocorticism, occurring in 80-85% of cases.

♥ Polyphagia is found in 60-90% of cases.

✓ Pendulous abdomen due to muscle weakness, obesity, and hepatomegaly in 70-90% (Figure 5-1).

✓ Redistribution of fat to the trunk results in truncal obesity.

✓ Cutaneous abnormalities are common with alopecia present in about 60%.

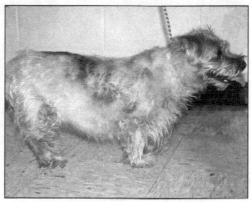

Figure 5-1 Dog with hyperadrenocorticism showing pendulous abdomen, truncal alopecia, and cutaneous hyperpigmentation.

✓ Alopecia is usually bilaterally symmetrical and truncal in distribution (Figure 5-2).

✓ Thin skin results in subcutaneous veins being readily visible in some dogs (Figure 5-3).

✓ Comedones, pyoderma, hyperpigmentation, and calcinosis cutis are sometimes present (see Figure 5-3).

✓ Lethargy is a frequent complaint.

✓ Mild weakness is common, and may be associated with muscle wasting and atrophy.

✓ Rarely, pseudomyotonia occurs, manifest by hypertonia that can be so severe that the limbs are stiff and the dog is unable to ambulate.

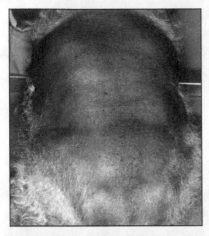

Figure 5-2 Miniature Poodle with pituitary-dependent hyperadrenocorticism. Note truncal obesity and bilaterally symmetrical alopecia sparing the limbs.

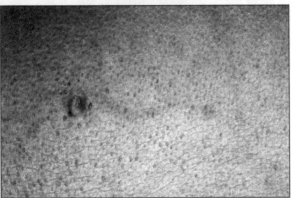

Figure 5-3 Thin skin with visible subcutaneous blood vessels and comedones in the dog in Figure 5-2.

✓ Excessive panting is common.

✓ Pulmonary mineralization with hypoxemia can occur in some cases.

✓ Pulmonary thromboembolism occurs occasionally resulting in an acute onset of respiratory distress, severe hypoxemia, and potentially death.

✓ Hypertension is frequently present in dogs with hyperadrenocorticism and specific treatment for this complication should be considered if the blood pressure is markedly elevated or does not normalize after resolution of the hyperadrenocorticism.

✓ Generalized hepatomegaly is palpable on physical examination in 70% of cases.

✓ Testicular atrophy and anestrus are common in intact animals.

✓ Neurological abnormalities including behavior changes, obtundation, disorientation, seizures, ataxia, pacing, tetraparesis, wide fluctuations in body temperature, blindness, and central vestibular signs can indicate a large pituitary tumor (macroadenoma).

Routine Laboratory Tests

✓ A stress leukogram is often present in hyperadrenocorticism, but is a nonspecific finding.

✓ The hematocrit may be high normal or slightly elevated.

♥ Serum alkaline phosphatase activity is elevated in 85-90% of dogs with hyperadrenocorticism; the elevations are often marked. The steroid isoenzyme of alkaline phosphatase is induced by cortisol and other corticosteroids in hyperadrenocorticism.

✓ Alanine aminotransferase (ALT) is frequently mildly to moderately elevated.

✓ Hypercholesterolemia is found in most affected dogs.

✓ Hyperglycemia and hypophosphatemia are occasionally present; diabetes mellitus may result from prolonged hyperadrenocorticism.

♥ Hyposthenuria or isosthenuria occurs in over 80% of dogs due to inhibition of the action of antidiuretic hormone on the renal collecting ducts (a form of acquired nephrogenic diabetes insipidus) and impaired secretion of antidiuretic hormone.

♥ Urinary tract infection is found in nearly 50% of dogs with hyperadrenocorticism. Clinical signs of urinary tract infection are usually absent in affected dogs. Pyuria and bacteriuria are absent in 40% and 30% of cases with infection, respectively.

✋ Urine culture should be performed in all animals with hyperadrenocorticism.

✓ Proteinuria is relatively common in dogs with hyperadrenocorticism and is renal in origin although the exact etiology is unknown.

Diagnostic Imaging

Abdominal imaging is useful in distinguishing PDH and adrenal tumors.

Abdominal radiographs

♥ Adrenal tumors are visible on routine abdominal radiographs in approximately 50% of cases of adrenal-dependent hyperadrenocorticism.

✓ Mineralization of adrenal tumors occurs in about 50% of both adenomas and adenocarcinomas.

✓ Hepatomegaly is usually present.

Thoracic Radiographs

✓ Diffuse pulmonary mineralization can be found.

✓ Pulmonary thromboembolism may result in an interstitial or alveolar pulmonary pattern, pleural effusion, regional hypoperfusion visualized as a hyperlucent area, enlarged pulmonary arteries, and/or cardiomegaly.

✓ Pulmonary metastases from adrenal adenocarcinomas are occasionally visualized.

Abdominal ultrasound

♥ Bilateral adrenomegaly or normal adrenal size is expected with PDH, while unilateral adrenomegaly is present in dogs with adrenal tumors.

✓ The normal right adrenal gland is V-shaped while the normal left adrenal gland is peanut-shaped when imaged in the transverse plane (Figure 5-4).

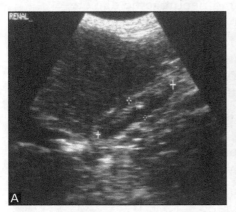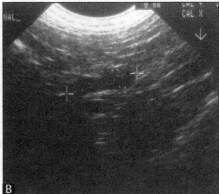

Figure 5-4 Ultrasound appearance of left and right adrenal glands in a normal dog. In the transverse plane, the right adrenal gland is V-shaped or cylindrical **(A)** and the left adrenal gland has a bilobed, peanut shape **(B)**.

✓ The maximum diameter of normal adrenal glands generally does not exceed 8 mm, but normal large dogs have been reported to have glands up to 12 mm. The glands should be measured at their largest diameter (not length).

♥ Adrenal glands maintain normal shape in most cases of PDH, although nodular hyperplasia is sometimes present (Figure 5-5).

♥ Adrenal tumors are identified as unilateral adrenal gland enlargement; the contralateral adrenal gland may be smaller than normal due to atrophy (Figure 5-6).

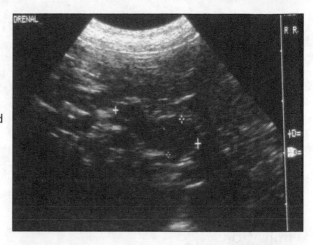

Figure 5-5 Enlarged left adrenal gland in a dog with pituitary-dependent hyperadrenocorticism. Normal shape is maintained but the corticomedullary distinction is lost and the adrenal gland is wider than normal.

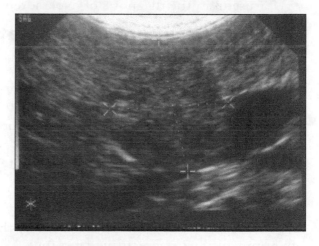

Figure 5-6 Right adrenal gland adenoma in an 11 yr Boston Terrier with hyperadrenocorticism.

✓ Concurrent adrenal tumor and PDH should be considered when one adrenal gland is greatly enlarged or asymmetrically enlarged while the contralateral gland is enlarged but of normal shape. This is very rare.

Screening Tests for Diagnosis of Hyperadrenocorticism

♥ Testing for hyperadrenocorticism occurs in two steps. First, a diagnosis of hyperadrenocorticism is made using a screening test. After the diagnosis has been established, discriminatory testing is used to determine if the hyperadrenocorticism is caused by an adrenal tumor or is pituitary-dependent.

Basal Cortisol Concentration

Overview

✓ Plasma cortisol concentrations fluctuate in normal dogs and in dogs with hyperadrenocorticism.

✓ Basal plasma cortisol concentrations are within the normal range in most dogs with hyperadrenocorticism, while dogs undergoing stress may have elevated plasma cortisol concentrations.

Interpretation

♥ No useful interpretation of basal cortisol concentrations can be made.

Limitations

✓ Not useful in the diagnosis of hyperadrenocorticism.

Urine Cortisol:creatinine Ratio

Overview

✓ The amount of cortisol in the urine is proportional to the plasma concentration over the period of time that the urine was formed.

♥ Very sensitive test that is positive in almost all dogs with hyperadrenocorticism.

♥ Specificity is low as any stress can elevate urine cortisol:creatinine ratio

Protocol

⚷ Urine samples should be collected by the owner in the home environment on 2 consecutive mornings.

✓ The samples should be refrigerated until submitted to the laboratory. Equal quantities of urine from the 2 samples are combined and submitted as a single sample for analysis. Alternatively, a single urine sample could be used.

Interpretation

✓ Elevated urine cortisol:creatinine ratio would be expected in all dogs with hyperadrenocorticism.

✋ A normal result rarely is found in hyperadrenocorticism.

✓ A positive test result indicates that hyperadrenocorticism is possible and that further testing is necessary to distinguish hyperadrenocorticism from stress-induced hypercortisolemia.

Limitations

💣 Urine cortisol:creatinine ratio is usually elevated in dogs with nonadrenal illness and in dogs stressed by examination and hospitalization.

♥ Urine samples must be collected at home for valid results.

ACTH response test

Overview

✔ Excellent first-line test for diagnosis of hyperadrenocorticism.

✔ Less affected by stress and nonadrenal illness than other tests.

✔ Less sensitive than other tests, particularly in dogs with adrenal tumors.

✔ Bioactivity of ACTH gel preparations is variable, so synthetic ACTH is recommended for testing.

Protocol

✔ Obtain blood sample for measurement of cortisol before and 1 hour after administration of synthetic ACTH at 5 µg/kg IV or IM.

✔ Reconstituted synthetic ACTH will remain active when frozen in plastic syringes for 6 months.

✔ Compounded ACTH gels result in variable times to peak cortisol concentration, so sampling at 1 and 2 hours post administration of 2.2 µ/kg of ACTH gel is indicated.

✔ Adrenocortical steroid hormones other than cortisol (17-hydroxyprogesterone or progesterone) can be measured in cases where cortisol concentrations are normal and hyperadrenocorticism is still considered likely. These hormones may be elevated in both PDH and adrenal tumors.

Interpretation

♥ Post-ACTH cortisol concentration elevated above the normal range is diagnostic of hyperadrenocorticism, but can also occur in dogs with nonadrenal illness.

✔ Not all dogs with hyperadrenocorticism will have an abnormal test.

✔ The normal range varies between laboratories; in general, normal basal cortisol concentrations are 0.5-4.0 µg/dl and normal post-ACTH cortisol is 8-20 µg/dl.

✔ Dogs with iatrogenic hyperadrenocorticism will have little to no increase in cortisol after ACTH administration.

Limitations

♥ Normal results are found in 40-60% of dogs with adrenocortical tumors and 5-15% of dogs with PDH.

✓ Does not distinguish between PDH and adrenal tumor.

Low-dose Dexamethasone Suppression Test (LDDS Test)

Overview

✓ Administration of dexamethasone normally reduces ACTH secretion via negative feedback to the pituitary gland. A subsequent decrease in plasma cortisol concentration occurs (Figure 5-7).

✓ Dogs with hyperadrenocorticism are resistant to this negative feedback and do not have suppression of cortisol.

♥ Excellent screening test because of its high sensitivity in diagnosing hyperadrenocorticism.

♥ Not as specific as the ACTH response test; false positive results are common in dogs that are ill with diseases not associated with hyperadrenocorticism.

Protocol

✓ Obtain blood samples for measurement of cortisol before and 4 and 8 hours after IV administration of 0.01 mg/kg dexamethasone.

✓ Dexamethasone sodium phosphate or dexamethasone in propylene glycol can both be used. Dexamethasone usually has to be diluted with sterile saline (1:10) for sufficiently accurate dosing.

Interpretation

✓ A normal response is suppression of cortisol concentrations below 1.0-1.5 µg/dl at both 4 and 8 hours after dexamethasone administration.

✓ A diagnosis of hyperadrenocorticism is made when the cortisol concentration on the 8-hour sample is above 1.5 µg/dl, although this can also occur in dogs with nonadrenal illness.

♥ If hyperadrenocorticism is diagnosed based on clinical signs and an elevated plasma cortisol concentration on the 8-hour sample, PDH can be differentiated from adrenal tumor in about 50% of cases.

A plasma cortisol concentration on the 4 or 8-hour post-dexamethasone sample that suppressed by greater than 50% of the baseline level is diagnostic of PDH.

PDH is also diagnosed if the 4-hour post-dexamethasone sample is less than 1.5 µg/dl and "escapes" at 8 hours (cortisol > 15 µg/dl).

Limitations

✓ Normal results are found in 5-10% of dogs with PDH and only very rarely in dogs with adrenal tumors.

✓ Iatrogenic hyperadrenocorticism cannot be diagnosed with the LDDS test.

♥ The specificity of the LDDS test is relatively low with over 50% of dogs with nonadrenal illness having an abnormal test result.

🖐 The LDDS test should only be used when there is a high suspicion of hyperadrenocorticism and concurrent illness is not present.

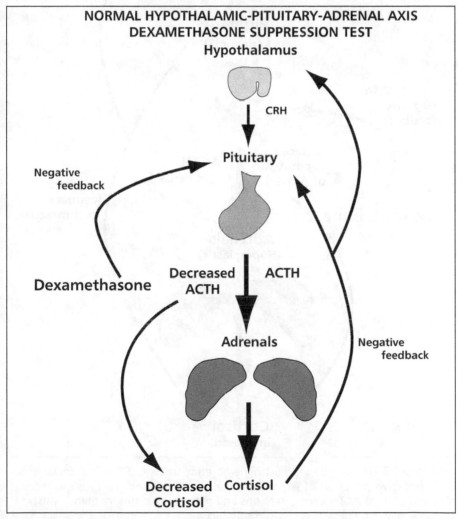

Figure 5-7A Administration of dexamethasone to a normal dog results in negative feedback that decreases pituitary secretion of ACTH. This results in a rapid and persistent decrease in plasma cortisol.

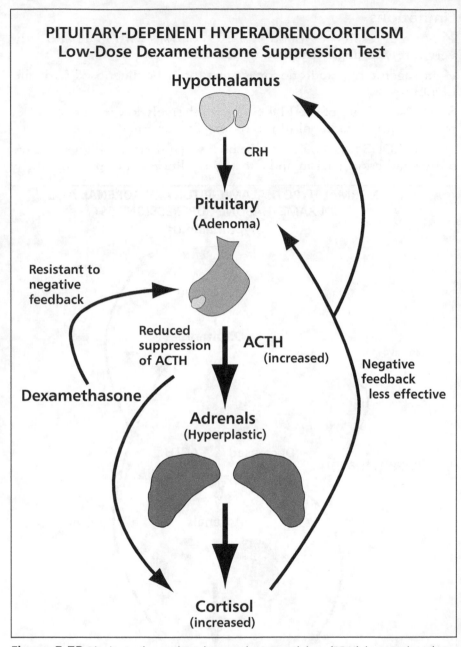

PITUITARY-DEPENENT HYPERADRENOCORTICISM
Low-Dose Dexamethasone Suppression Test

Hypothalamus

CRH

Pituitary
(Adenoma)

Resistant to
negative
feedback

Reduced
suppression
of ACTH

ACTH
(increased)

Negative
feedback
less effective

Dexamethasone

Adrenals
(Hyperplastic)

Cortisol
(increased)

Figure 5-7B Pituitary-dependent hyperadrenocorticism (PDH) is associated
with excessive secretion of ACTH from the pituitary gland. This results in
elevated plasma ACTH concentrations and makes the pituitary gland resistant
to suppression by low doses of dexamethasone.

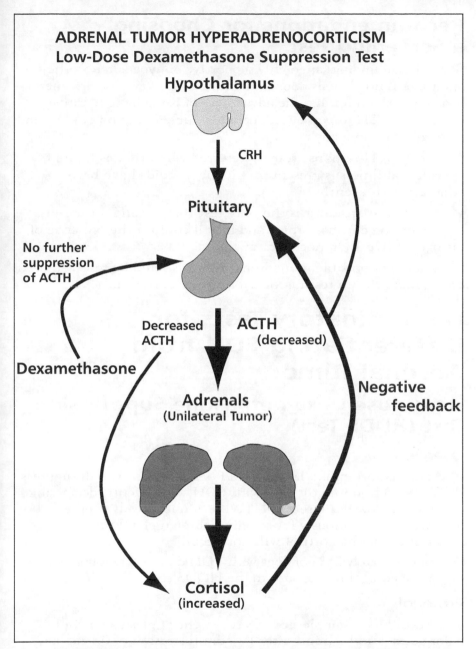

Figure 5-7C Adrenal tumor induced hyperadrenocorticism is caused by an autonomously functioning adrenal tumor. The cortisol secreted by this tumor reduces ACTH secretion through a negative feedback mechanism, resulting in decreased plasma ACTH concentrations. Administration of dexamethasone at any dose will not cause further suppression of ACTH secretion and will not suppress plasma cortisol levels.

Recommendations for Choosing a Screening Test

♥ If clinical findings are highly supportive of hyperadrenocorticism and there is no obvious nonadrenal illness, the low-dose dexamethasone suppression test has the advantages of being more sensitive than the ACTH response test and allows differentiation of PDH and adrenal tumor in many cases.

♥ The ACTH response test is preferred when time is limited, nonadrenal illness is present, or glucocorticoids have been administered recently.

✔ ACTH response test is the only test that is valid for use in a dog receiving corticosteroids and it will confirm the presence of iatrogenic hyperadrenocorticism.

♥ Whenever possible, nonadrenal illness should be resolved or controlled prior to testing for hyperadrenocorticism.

Discriminatory Tests for Differentiating PDH from Adrenal Tumor

High-dose Dexamethasone Suppression Test (HDDS Test)

Overview

✔ Administration of a large dose of dexamethasone will suppress ACTH secretion in most dogs with PDH, subsequently decreasing plasma cortisol. Because ACTH secretion is already suppressed in dogs with autonomously functioning adrenal gland tumors, suppression of plasma cortisol will not occur.

♥ Approximately 25% of dogs with PDH do not have suppression of plasma cortisol in response to the HDDS test.

Protocol

✔ Obtain blood samples for measurement of plasma cortisol before and 4 and 8 hours after IV administration of 0.1 mg/kg dexamethasone.

Interpretation

♥ Suppression of plasma cortisol to less than 50% of the baseline concentration or a decrease in plasma cortisol to less than 1.5 μg/dl on either the 4 or 8-hour sample is diagnostic of PDH.

✔ It is extremely rare for suppression of cortisol to occur in a dog with an adrenal tumor.

✔ Failure of cortisol to suppress occurs in both PDH and adrenal tumors, and further testing is necessary to determine the cause of hyperadrenocorticism.

Limitations

♥ Differentiation of PDH and adrenal tumors occurs only if suppression of cortisol occurs.

✔ The HDDS test is not diagnostic in approximately 40% of cases because failure to suppress could indicate either adrenal tumor or PDH.

Endogenous Plasma ACTH Concentration

Overview

✔ PDH is caused by excessive production of ACTH by the pituitary gland while adrenal tumors produce cortisol autonomously that then causes negative feedback and suppresses ACTH secretion. Plasma ACTH concentration is elevated in PDH and below normal in dogs with adrenal tumors (Figure 5-7).

Protocol

✔ Obtain blood sample in appropriate anticoagulant (usually EDTA) preferably in a plastic tube.

✋ Sample must be handled properly for results to be valid. The sample must be placed on ice, centrifuged, and stored frozen in a plastic tube since ACTH will adhere to glass.

✔ If shipped to a laboratory, the sample must arrive frozen, so dry ice may be necessary for transport.

✔ Aprotinin is a protease inhibitor that will dramatically reduce degradation of ACTH; its use (in tubes provided by the reference laboratory) can simplify collection and transport.

Interpretation

✔ Adrenal tumor is confirmed by finding a plasma ACTH concentration below the normal range (usually < 20 pg/ml).

✔ PDH is confirmed by a plasma ACTH concentration above the normal range (usually > 40-45 pg/ml).

Limitations

✔ As many as 40% of samples for measurement of plasma ACTH are nondiagnostic.

✓ Measurement of ACTH in more than one sample will increase the accuracy of the test; blood samples can be obtained 30-60 minutes apart. If one or both of the samples have a plasma ACTH concentration below or above the normal range, a specific diagnosis can be made.

Abdominal Radiographs and Ultrasound

✓ As discussed above, diagnostic imaging can be an excellent tool to discriminate PDH and adrenal tumor.

♥ Abdominal ultrasonography in the hands of an experienced operator may be the most consistently accurate method of identifying adrenal tumors and is the test of choice in the authors' practices.

Treatment Recommendations

✋ Not all dogs with hyperadrenocorticism need to be treated at the time of diagnosis.

✓ The benefits of treatment in dogs without significant clinical signs or complications must be weighed with the potential complications and costs of treatment.

✓ Dogs with a combination of significant PU/PD, recurrent urinary tract infections, cutaneous manifestations, diabetes mellitus, and other clinical signs or complications should be treated.

✓ If treatment is delayed, owners should be warned of possible complications including hypertension, diabetes mellitus, infection, pulmonary thromboembolism, glomerular disease, and pancreatitis.

Mitotane (o,p'-DDD)

✓ Mitotane is an adrenocorticolytic drug that selectively destroys the zonas reticularis and fasciculata of the adrenal cortex, sparing the zona glomerulosa and thus aldosterone secretion in most cases.

✓ Treatment consists of induction and maintenance phases.

💣 Side effects can be life threatening and owners should be made aware of the clinical signs associated with mitotane-induced side effects.

✓ Can be effective for treatment of both PDH and adrenal tumors.

Objectives

✓ Relieve clinical signs of hyperadrenocorticism and minimize complications of the disease by inducing atrophy and necrosis of the adrenal cortex.

✓ Reduce cortisol secretion such that plasma cortisol concentrations are within the normal <u>resting</u> range before and after ACTH administration using the induction phase of treatment.

✓ Do not suppress aldosterone secretion with treatment.

✓ Maintain suppressed cortisol secretion during maintenance treatment.

Treatment Protocol for PDH

Induction Treatment

✓ Administer mitotane at 25 mg/kg orally twice per day.

🖑 Administer mitotane with food as fat increases absorption considerably.

💣 Continue treatment until one of the following occurs:

7 days of treatment have been administered.

Water consumption has decreased to < 60 ml/kg/day.

Food consumption has substantially decreased.

Clinical signs of side effects develop.

♥ An ACTH response test should be performed at the end of induction treatment.

💣 No further mitotane treatment is administered until the results of the ACTH response test are evaluated.

♥ If the post-ACTH plasma cortisol concentration is within the normal <u>resting</u> range (1.0-4.0 µg/dl), maintenance treatment is initiated.

♥ If the post-ACTH cortisol is not adequately suppressed, further induction treatment should be administered at the same dose for an additional 2-5 days. The above monitoring parameters should be followed and another ACTH response test should be performed at the end of treatment.

✓ Induction treatment may have to be repeated if clinical signs or hypercortisolemia occurs during maintenance treatment.

Maintenance Treatment

✓ Begin maintenance treatment following successful induction treatment.

✓ The dosage and timing of maintenance treatment with mitotane is dependent on the response during induction treatment.

If induction treatment is successful after 5 or fewer days of treatment, a maintenance dose of 25 mg/kg weekly should be administered.

If induction treatment is required for 6 days or longer before post-ACTH cortisol concentration is adequately suppressed, a maintenance dose of 50 mg/kg/week is indicated.

Maintenance dosage can be split into 2-3 doses based on ease of administration of the 500 mg tablets.

✓ If clinical signs of hyperadrenocorticism recur or if the post-ACTH cortisol concentration is above the resting range, another course of daily induction mitotane treatment must be instituted.

The duration of this treatment depends on the clinical picture, but 25 mg/kg twice daily for 3-7 days is recommended.

Some dogs will require a higher dose of mitotane during this induction period, particularly when repeated induction treatments have been administered.

The dosage of mitotane for maintenance treatment must be increased by 25-50% subsequent to the repeat induction treatment.

Treatment Protocol for Adrenal Tumors

✓ Mitotane administration to dogs with adrenal tumors destroys neoplastic adrenal tissue.

✓ Mitotane can be used as the sole treatment for adrenal tumors or as an adjunct to surgery to alleviate the negative effects of hyperadrenocorticism and reduce the tumor size prior to attempted adrenalectomy.

✓ Treatment is similar to that for PDH except the mitotane dose is increased slightly and the duration of treatment is likely to be longer.

✓ The induction dose of mitotane should be 50-75 mg/kg total daily dose for 7-10 days. Additional induction treatment is frequently necessary to adequately suppress cortisol secretion.

✓ Monitoring of treatment, including side effects, resolution of clinical signs, and ACTH response tests is identical to that for treatment of PDH.

Monitoring Treatment with Mitotane

Induction Treatment

♥ Owners should be instructed verbally and in writing the criteria for cessation of mitotane treatment and the side effects of the drug. It is recommended that the owner be contacted daily during induction treatment to identify response to treatment and side effects in a timely manner.

♥ Decreases in water consumption and food intake in dogs with PU/PD and polyphagia generally indicate a response to treatment.

💣 Side effects include vomiting, anorexia, depression, diarrhea, and ataxia and are due to a rapid decrease in plasma cortisol.

✓ The most severe side effect is hypoadrenocorticism with both glucocorticoid and mineralocorticoid deficiency. Serum electrolytes should be measured in dogs with significant side effects in order to determine if a mineralocorticoid deficiency is present.

✓ Side effects occur during the induction period in about 25% of dogs.

♥ Administration of prednisone at 0.4 mg/kg orally once per day will alleviate the clinical signs due to cortisol deficiency in some dogs.

💣 Owners of all dogs treated with mitotane should have prednisone available for use if side effects occur.

♥ Many dogs that develop side effects will require parenteral glucocorticoids and IV fluids since vomiting and dehydration are common.

♥ After the initial induction treatment is complete, an ACTH response test should be performed in each case.

✋ If the dog is receiving prednisone, a period of at least 24 hours should elapse between the ACTH response test and the previous prednisone administration.

♥ A post-ACTH cortisol concentration in the normal resting range (1.0-4.0 µg/dl) indicates adequate treatment and maintenance treatment should be initiated.

✓ A post-ACTH cortisol concentration above the normal resting range (> 4.0 µg/dl) indicates inadequate suppression of adrenocortical function and the need for further induction treatment.

✓ If further induction treatment is necessary, an ACTH response test is performed at the end of each course, and further treatment is determined as outlined above.

Maintenance Treatment

✓ Approximately 50% of dogs treated with mitotane for PDH will have a recurrence of clinical signs or a post-ACTH cortisol concentration above the normal resting range within 1 year of initial induction treatment.

✓ Response to mitotane treatment should be monitored by observing for recurrence of clinical signs of hyperadrenocorticism and monitoring ACTH response tests.

✔ ACTH response tests should be performed 1 month after induction treatment, then once every 6 months or anytime that clinical signs of hyperadrenocorticism recur.

✔ Further induction treatment should be instituted if the post-ACTH cortisol concentration is above the normal resting range as outlined above under maintenance treatment.

L-Deprenyl

✔ L-deprenyl (selegiline) is a monamine oxidase inhibitor that increases dopamine. Dopamine in the pituitary gland inhibits secretion of ACTH.

♥ Effective only for dogs with PDH; no effect in dogs with adrenal tumors.

♥ The efficacy of L-deprenyl is variable and inconsistent.

✋ Dogs with severe signs of hyperadrenocorticism should be treated with another drug since L-deprenyl may be effective in as few as 10-20% of cases.

Objectives

✔ Relieve clinical signs of hyperadrenocorticism, presumably through reduction in hypercortisolemia.

Treatment Protocol

✔ Administer L-deprenyl at an initial dose of 1 mg/kg once daily for 2 months. Increase the dose to 2 mg/kg once daily if clinical improvement is not noted within 2 months at the lower dosage.

✔ If no response is noted within 1 month of initiating the higher dose of L-deprenyl or if clinical signs of hyperadrenocorticism are progressive during treatment, an alternative treatment should be instituted.

Monitoring Treatment

✔ No objective method of monitoring treatment has been defined.

✔ Success of treatment is determined by relief of clinical signs including reduction of PU, PD, polyphagia, panting, increased level of activity, improvement in dermatologic abnormalities, pendulous abdomen, and hepatomegaly.

✔ Improvement in these clinical signs may be due to effects of L-deprenyl independent of those reducing plasma cortisol concentrations.

✔ Urine cortisol:creatinine ratio would be expected to decrease in dogs where excessive cortisol secretion is controlled and this test may be useful in monitoring treatment.

✓ Side effects of treatment are uncommon and include hyperactivity, agitation, vomiting, anorexia, ataxia, and disorientation.

✓ Hypoadrenocorticism and associated hyperkalemia and hyponatremia will not occur as a side effect of L-deprenyl.

✓ Adverse drug interactions have not been evaluated in dogs, but drugs to be avoided in dogs receiving L-deprenyl include other monoamine oxidase inhibitors, tricyclic antidepressants (amitriptyline), fluoxeitine, other antidepressants, ephedrine, and meperidine and other opioids.

Ketoconazole

✓ Inhibits adrenal steroid synthesis thus decreasing secretion of cortisol and other adrenal-derived steroids.

✓ Effective in treatment of both PDH and adrenal tumors.

✓ About 20-25% of dogs do not respond to ketoconazole treatment.

✓ Can be administered for long-term management of dogs that do not tolerate mitotane.

✓ More expensive than most of the other treatment options.

Objectives

✓ Suppress cortisol production and secretion.

✓ Useful for temporary treatment of adrenal tumors prior to surgery as well as long-term management of PDH.

✓ Onset of action is rapid, with a reduction in plasma cortisol occurring within hours of administration of a single dose.

Treatment Protocol

✓ Administer at 5 mg/kg twice daily for 7 days.

✓ Increase dose to 10 mg/kg twice daily if no adverse effects (vomiting, icterus) are noted.

✓ Dosage can be increased up to 15-20 mg/kg twice daily as necessary to control clinical signs and reduce the post-ACTH cortisol concentration.

Monitoring Treatment

✓ Monitor response to treatment by assessing clinical signs and ACTH response test 14 days after initiating treatment.

✓ Maintain post-ACTH cortisol concentration at less than 5.0 µg/dl.

✓ Side effects of ketoconazole include vomiting, anorexia, and reversible hepatotoxicity.

✓ Absorption may be decreased when administered concurrently with drugs that inhibit gastric acid secretion.

Trilostane

✓ Inhibits adrenal steroid enzyme activity, decreasing secretion of cortisol and other adrenal corticosteroids.

✓ Effective in treatment of both PDH and adrenal tumors.

✓ Appears to be a safe and effective drug. May become the preferred treatment if trilostane becomes widely available.

✓ More expensive than many other treatments.

Objectives

✓ Suppress cortisol and other corticosteroid production and secretion.

✓ Useful for long-term management of PDH and possibly adrenal tumors.

Treatment Protocol

✓ Dosages have not been well defined due to limited capsule sizes.

✓ Administer once daily at 30 mg for dogs less than 5 kg body weight, 60 mg for dogs 5-20 kg, and 120 mg for dogs weighing more than 20 kg.

✓ Dosage can be adjusted based on the clinical response and results of ACTH response testing.

Monitoring Treatment

✓ Perform an ACTH response test after 14 days of treatment. The test should be preformed within 4-6 hours of trilostane administration as its duration of effect appears to be less than 24 hours.

✓ Post-ACTH plasma cortisol concentration should be less than 5.0 µg/dl.

♥ Side effects are uncommon and appear to primarily result from overdosage, with subsequent hypoadrenocorticism including hyperkalemia and hyponatremia.

While the hypoadrenocorticism is usually reversible with cessation of trilostane administration, adrenal gland necrosis can occur. In these cases aggressive treatment is necessary to address the severe electrolyte disturbances and cortisol deficiency. Prolonged remission of hyperadrenocorticism following discontinuation of trilostane treatment is likely to occur in these cases, although clinical signs of hyperadrenocorticism recur in many cases.

Treatment of Pituitary Macroadenoma

✓ Macroadenomas can cause serious and progressive neurological signs.

✓ External beam radiation treatment is the only effective treatment.

✓ Most dogs will have either improvement or no progression of their neurologic deficits after treatment.

✓ Many dogs require treatment with mitotane or another drug to control signs of hyperadrenocorticism after radiation therapy.

✓ Median survival after pituitary irradiation is approximately 1 year.

✓ Prognosis is related to severity of neurological signs.

Management of Concurrent Diabetes Mellitus and Hyperadrenocorticism

✓ Hyperadrenocorticism results in insulin resistance and can cause diabetes mellitus.

💣* Treatment of the hyperadrenocorticism will result in a decrease in insulin requirements and increase the risk of hypoglycemia.

♥ Prior to treatment in a dog where the hyperglycemia is reasonably well controlled, the dosage of insulin should be reduced by 10-25%.

♥ Owners should monitor urine glucose daily during induction treatment with mitotane and the dosage of insulin reduced by an additional 20-25% if it is negative.

✓ The treatment protocol using mitotane, ketoconazole, or trilostane is not altered in diabetic dogs.

✓ Administration of prednisone at 0.2 mg/kg once daily is recommended during induction. Prednisone should be withdrawn for at least 24 hours before performing an ACTH response test.

✓ At the time the ACTH response test is performed to monitor response to mitotane treatment, a blood glucose curve should be performed to determine if an adjustment in the insulin dose is necessary. The ACTH response test should be performed at the end of the day.

✓ Control of the diabetes mellitus is again assessed approximately 4 weeks after completion of induction treatment and the insulin dosage is adjusted as necessary. Continued monitoring of urine glucose during this 4 weeks is recommended to avoid a hypoglycemic crisis.

✓ A small percentage of dogs no longer require insulin after controlling the hyperadrenocorticism, while the majority remain diabetic but are more easily controlled on a lower dose of insulin.

Surgical Management of Adrenal Tumors

✓ Adrenalectomy is the optimal treatment in some dogs with unilateral adrenal tumors.

✓ Considerable effort should be made to ensure that gross metasatasis or invasion of surrounding structures such as the caudal vena cava has not occurred prior to surgery.

✓ Perioperative complications are common and include sepsis, thromboembolism, pancreatitis, and hypoadrenocorticism. The mortality rate associated with surgery and the immediate post-operative period is 20-25%.

✓ Intensive management and surgical experience are necessary to optimize outcome.

Prognosis

✓ The duration of survival of dogs with untreated hyperadrenocorticism is unknown.

✓ The mean survival of dogs with hyperadrenocorticism treated with mitotane is 2 to 2.5 years, with many dogs dying of unrelated diseases.

✓ Successful complete resection of adrenal tumors is curative unless metastasis has occurred.

Feline Hyperadrenocorticism

♥ **Problems**

Alopecia

Thin skin

Fragile skin

Pendulous abdomen

Hepatomegaly

Diabetes mellitus

Polyuria

Polydipsia

Polyphagia

Obesity

Weakness

Muscle wasting

Hyperglycemia

Isosthenuria

Recurrent or persistent infections

Elevated liver enzymes

Hypercholesterolemia

Overview

✔ Hyperadrenocorticism is a rare disorder in older cats.

♥ Diabetes mellitus is usually present secondary to the hyperadrenocorticism.

✔ Adrenal tumors account for approximately 20% of cases and pituitary-dependent hyperadrenocorticism makes up 80% of the disease in cats. The occurrence of adenomas and carcinomas are approximately equal.

✔ Many cats with hyperadrenocorticism have advanced disease and are quite debilitated.

✔ Progesterone secreting adrenal tumors have been reported to cause clinical signs of hyperadrenocorticism.

Clinical Signs

✔ Polyuria, polydipsia, and polyphagia are the most common clinical signs and result at least in part because of concurrent diabetes mellitus found in most cats diagnosed with hyperadrenocorticism. These signs can occur in the absence of diabetes mellitus.

✔ A history of poorly controlled diabetes mellitus with or without insulin resistance is common.

✔ Weight gain and obesity are present in about 50% of cases despite the presence of diabetes mellitus. Weight loss occurs in some cats.

✔ Pendulous abdomen is usually present (Figure 5-8).

✔ Thin skin with visible subcutaneous blood vessels that is very fragile is often found. Routine restraint and grooming can cause large tears in the skin that heal slowly (Figure 5-9).

✔ Patchy alopecia, slow hair regrowth after clipping, and seborrhea may be found (Figure 5-10).

✔ Infections, including cystitis, pneumonia, abcesses, cutaneous infections, demodicosis, and others can be present.

✔ Hepatomegaly secondary to fatty infiltration from the diabetes mellitus as well as steroid hepatopathy is common.

✔ Clinical signs are often present for many months prior to diagnosis.

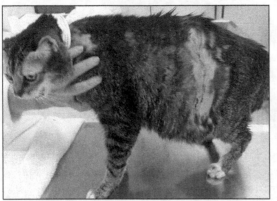

Figure 5-8
Cat with pituitary-dependent hyperadrenocorticism. Note pendulous abdomen and healing laceration that occurred with minimal trauma 6 weeks previously.

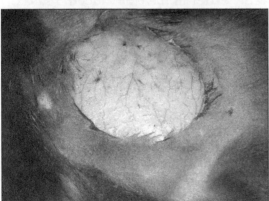

Figure 5-9
Laceration that occurred without known trauma in a cat with iatrogenic hyperadreno-corticism.

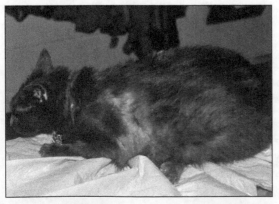

Figure 5-10
Alopecia and seborrhea in a cat with hyperadrenocorticism.

Routine Laboratory Tests

♥ Hyperglycemia is the most common biochemical abnormality as most cats are diabetic when a diagnosis of hyperadrenocorticism is made. Mild hyperglycemia is usually present in cats without overt diabetes mellitus.

✓ Elevated liver enzyme activity is common, but the elevations of alkaline phosphatase are much smaller in the cat than in the dog. Elevated liver enzymes can occur in the absence of diabetes mellitus.

✓ Hypercholesterolemia is found in over 50% of cases.

Diagnostic Imaging

✓ Adrenomegaly may be found on abdominal radiographs of some cats with adrenal gland neoplasia.

✓ Normal cats (up to 30%) can have mineralization of the adrenal glands, so adrenal mineralization is not an indication of hyperadrenocorticism or adrenal neoplasia.

✓ Hepatomegaly is common.

♥ Abdominal ultrasound can identify unilateral adrenomegaly in cats with adrenal tumors or bilateral adrenomegaly in many cats with PDH.

♥ Computed tomography (CT) of the pituitary may reveal a pituitary tumor, although not all cats with hyperadrenocorticism will have a visible tumor. CT is a useful tool for evaluating cats with an unknown cause of insulin resistant diabetes mellitus.

Tests for Diagnosis of Hyperadrenocorticism

Urine Cortisol: Creatinine Ratio

Overview

✓ Appears to be a sensitive test for cats with hyperadrenocorticism, but may have poor specificity.

Protocol

✓ Obtain urine at home using nonabsorbent litter such as aquarium gravel, preferably on 2 consecutive days. Samples should be refrigerated until analysis and equal quantities of urine can be mixed and submitted together for analysis.

Interpretation

♥ A normal urine cortisol:creatinine ratio makes hyperadrenocorticism very unlikely.

♥ A positive test is an indication for further testing of adrenal function.

Limitations

♥ Cats with nonadrenal illness frequently have elevated urine cortisol:creatinine ratio, so the specificity of the test is low.

ACTH Response Test

Overview

♥ Results are diagnostic of hyperadrenocorticism in most cases.

✓ Can be affected by nonadrenal illness resulting in a false positive test.

Protocol

✓ Obtain blood for measurement of cortisol before and 1 and 2 hours after intravenous administration of 125 μg cosyntropin (synthetic ACTH).

✓ Alternatively, samples can be obtained 30 and 60 minutes after intramuscular administration of cosyntropin.

✓ Measurement of progesterone or 17-hydroxyprogesterone may be useful if the plasma cortisol response is normal and hyperadrenocorticism is still suspected.

Interpretation

✓ The peak plasma cortisol response to synthetic ACTH is variable, so the highest of the 2 post-ACTH cortisol concentrations should be chosen to interpret.

✓ The normal post-ACTH cortisol concentration is dependent on laboratory established ranges, but a range of 8-16 μg/dl is representative.

♥ A post-ACTH cortisol above 16 μg/dl is consistent with hyperadrenocorticism.

Limitations

✓ Normal results on ACTH stimulation testing occurs relatively commonly in cats with hyperadrenocorticism.

♥ Cats with nonadrenal illness may have a false positive test, including cats with diabetes mellitus.

Dexamethasone Suppression Test

Overview

✓ Plasma cortisol in normal cats is more resistant to suppression after dexamethasone administration than dogs. Therefore, a higher dose (0.1 mg/kg) is used for a screening test.

More sensitive than ACTH response test.

Protocol

✓ Obtain blood samples for measurement of cortisol before and 4 and 8 hours after administration of 0.1 mg/kg dexamethasone IV.

Interpretation

♥ Suppression of plasma cortisol concentration to <1.0 µg/dl is normal, while a post-dexamethasone cortisol concentration above 1.5 µg/dl is consistent with hyperadrenocorticism.

✓ Suppression of plasma cortisol by >50% of baseline on the 4 or 8-hour sample is consistent with pituitary-dependent hyperadrenocorticism.

Limitations

♥ Some cats with hyperadrenocorticism will have a normal response to dexamethasone suppression.

✓ Many cats with PDH will not suppress by >50 of baseline cortisol, so the dexamethasone suppression test is not a sensitive method for diagnosing PDH.

♥ The effects of nonadrenal illness are not well defined in cats, but it would be expected that false positive results will occur in some cats with normal adrenal function and unrelated illness.

Endogenous Plasma ACTH Concentration

Overview

✓ Use to differentiate PDH from adrenal tumor.

Protocol

✓ Obtain sample in EDTA and process immediately. Must be stored in a plastic tube and shipped frozen.

Interpretation

♥ Plasma ACTH concentrations in cats with PDH should be in the mid-normal or above normal range. Cats with adrenal tumors should have low or low-normal plasma ACTH.

✓ Appears to be an accurate test for discriminating between types of hyperadrenocorticism.

Limitations

⊶ Sample handling must be performed appropriately for valid results.

Treatment Recommendations

💣 Hyperadrenocorticism in cats will have serious consequences if left untreated.

✓ Diabetes mellitus may resolve in many cases or at least be easier to effectively manage after resolution of the hyperadrenocorticism.

♥ Medical management has not been consistently effective.

✓ The ideal treatment remains to be determined.

Adrenalectomy

♥ Bilateral adrenalectomy in cats with PDH and unilateral adrenalectomy in cats with adrenal tumors is reported to be the most successful treatment.

♥ Perioperative mortality rate is 25-30%.

Objectives

✓ Eliminate excessive glucocorticoid secretion.

Treatment Protocol

♥ Preoperative medical management may reduce the complications.

♥ Due to the high complication rate and the location of the adrenal glands, referral to an appropriately experienced surgical and medical team is recommended.

💣 Glucocorticoid supplementation is necessary for 1-2 months after unilateral adrenalectomy for an adrenal tumor.

💣 Bilateral adrenalectomy results in deficiencies of glucocorticoids and mineralocorticoids, so treatment with fludrocortisone or desoxycorticosterone pivalate and prednisone are required for the remainder of the cat's life.

Monitoring Treatment

♥ Cats with uncontrolled hyperadrenocorticism are at considerable risk for complications during and after surgery including infections, poor wound healing, pancreatitis, hypoglycemia due to insulin overdose, and thrombosis. Electrolyte disturbances are common in cats undergoing bilateral adrenalectomy.

✓ Intensive postoperative management is crucial to the success of adrenalectomy.

♥ Periodic evaluation of electrolytes should be performed in cats following bilateral adrenalectomy. Fatal hypoadrenocorticism can occur if treatment is inadequately monitored.

✓ Adjustment or elimination of insulin treatment will be necessary in cats with concurrent diabetes mellitus.

Mitotane

✓ Efficacy of mitotane is reported to be variable in feline hyperadrenocorticism and is unlikely to be effective in most cases.

Objectives

✓ Eliminate clinical signs of hyperadrenocorticism without inducing severe adrenocortical deficiency.

Treatment Protocol

Induction Treatment

♥ Identical to treatment of PDH in the dog.

✓ Mitotane at 25 mg/kg orally twice daily for 7 days.

♥ Stop treatment if side effects as described in the dog occur.

✓ Perform ACTH response test at the end of the 7-day treatment.

✓ Adequate treatment is evidenced by post-ACTH plasma cortisol concentration within the normal resting range (1-4 μg/dl).

✓ Repeated induction treatment may be necessary to control signs and adequately reduce cortisol secretion.

Maintenance Treatment

♥ Identical to dog.

Administer mitotane at 25 mg/kg twice per week.

✓ Monitor in 1 month, then every 6 months or when clinical signs return.

Monitoring Treatment

✓ ACTH response tests are used to determine if treatment has adequately suppressed adrenocortical function.

●✳ Clinical signs of hypoadrenocorticism include anorexia, vomiting, diarrhea, and weakness. Mitotane treatment should be stopped and prednisone (2.5 mg daily) should be administered if illness occurs. An ACTH response test and serum biochemistries including electrolytes should be performed if hypoadrenocorticism is suspected.

✔ Because mitotane treatment is often not effective, an alternative treatment should be sought if induction treatment is not successful after 14-21 days.

Metyrapone

✔ Metyrapone is an inhibitor of an adrenocortical enzyme involved in synthesis of cortisol.

♥ Response has been variable in the few cats reported, but this treatment is a viable option.

Objectives

✔ Suppress cortisol secretion sufficiently to reduce or eliminate clinical signs of hyperadrenocorticism.

Treatment Protocol

✔ Administer metyrapone at 30-50 mg/kg orally twice daily.

Monitoring Treatment

✔ Clinical signs should improve or resolve on treatment.

✔ ACTH response tests can be used to monitor efficacy of treatment, although improvement in clinical signs without control of cortisol levels has been reported.

✔ Side effects may occur related to excessive suppression of cortisol synthesis.

Ketoconazole

✔ Response to treatment has been variable, with many cats not responding adequately to treatment.

✔ Other drugs are probably more effective with fewer side effects.

Aminoglutethimide

✔ Aminoglutethimide is an adrenal steroid enzyme inhibitor that blocks synthesis of most adrenocortical steroids.

♥ Safe in the limited number of cats reported, although clinical signs may not completely resolve or may recur during treatment.

Objectives

✔ Suppress cortisol secretion sufficiently to reduce or eliminate clinical signs of hyperadrenocorticism.

Treatment Protocol

✔ Administer aminoglutethimide at 6 mg/kg twice daily.

✔ Experience with the drug is limited, but side effects have not been noted

Monitoring Treatment

✔ Clinical response and ACTH response tests are used to monitor response to treatment. The post-ACTH cortisol concentration should be in the normal <u>resting</u> range.

Trilostane

✔ Inhibitor of adrenal steroid enzyme activity.

✔ There is limited experience using trilostane in cats, and it appears less consistently effective than when used in dogs.

✔ Safety of trilostane in cats is unknown.

Objectives

✔ Suppress secretion of cortisol and other steroid hormones.

✔ May be useful in long-term management of hyperadrenocorticism.

Treatment Protocol

✔ Administer orally at 30 mg once daily. Adjust dosage to maintain post-ACTH cortisol below 5-7 µg/dl.

✔ Twice daily treatment may improve the clinical response.

Monitoring Treatment

✔ Monitor clinical signs and ACTH response tests.

✔ Overdosage may result in hypoadrenocorticism.

Limitations

✔ Incomplete response appears to commonly occur during trilostane administration in cats.

✔ Not approved for use in North America.

Prognosis

♥ The prognosis is poor without treatment; infections, poorly-regulated diabetes mellitus, thromboembolism, skin lacerations, heart failure and other complications result in death in inadequately treated cats.

♥ Adequate treatment such as adrenalectomy can result in long-term survival.

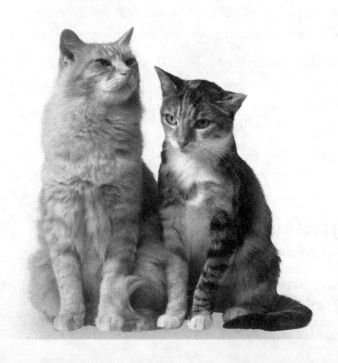

Section 6

Hypoadrenocorticism (Addison's Disease)

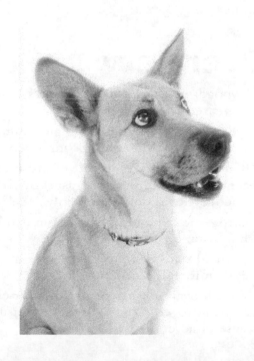

♥ Problems

Weakness

Lethargy

Vomiting

Hematemesis

Diarrhea

Dehydration

Hypothermia

Melena

Polyuria/Polydipsia

Hyperkalemia

Hyponatremia

Hypoalbuminemia

Anemia (non-regenerative)

Hypercalcemia

Azotemia with isosthenuria

Bradycardia

Hypotension

Shaking

Seizures

Shock

Overview

♥ Hypoadrenocorticism (Addison's Disease) can be a life-threatening emergency.

✓ Predominantly results from autoimmune destruction of the adrenal glands (primary hypoadrenocorticism).

✓ Rarely it can be the result of insufficient ACTH production (secondary hypoadrenocorticism) by the pituitary gland leading to glucocorticoid deficiency only.

✓ Iatrogenic hypoadrenocorticism can be induced by treatment with mitotane.

✓ Clinical signs develop because of a deficiency of glucocorticoids or mineralocorticoids or both.

✓ Withdrawal of corticosteroids after chronic treatment may result in iatrogenic hypoadrenocorticism (glucocorticoids only) because of adrenocortical atrophy.

✓ When glucocorticoids production alone is absent, it may also be termed atypical Addison's disease.

✓ A marked predisposition for young female dogs and certain breeds such as Standard Poodles, Great Danes, Portuguese Water Dogs, Bearded Collies, Rottweilers, West Highland White Terriers and Wheaten Terriers is present.

✓ Incidence is low, about 1 case per 3000 dogs.

✓ The disease does occur in cats but is rare.

Common Clinical Signs

Typical vs. Atypical Addison's

✓ The term atypical hypoadrenocorticism is applied when only glucocorticoid deficiency is present. This can be from secondary or primary hypoadrenocorticism. In some cases of primary hypoadrenocorticism the cells that produce glucocorticoids are affected before the cells that produce mineralocorticoids. Some cases will eventually develop mineralocorticoid deficiency as well.

✓ Mineralocorticoids play a vital role in regulating electrolytes and fluid balance. Without aldosterone (main adrenal mineralocorticoid) potassium is no longer excreted adequately while increased loss of sodium occurs. The lack of sodium results in inadequate circulating blood volume. This leads to a decrease in cardiac output and reduced perfusion of organs including the kidney. The renal medullary gradient is also "washed out" leading to a reduced ability to concentrate urine.

✓ Hypovolemia, hyperkalemia and hyponatremia and resultant signs occur secondary to mineralocorticoid deficiency.

✓ Glucocorticoid deficiency results in weakness, GI hemorrhage and hypoglycemia (decreased gluconeogenesis in the liver, increased insulin receptor sensitivity). In addition, hyponatremia may occur as a result of an impaired ability to excrete free water (ADH release is not counteracted by glucocorticoids).

General

✓ Because of the varied clinical signs present with hypoadrenocorticism it can be difficult to establish a diagnosis.

♥ A chronic illness, consisting of anorexia, lethargy, vomiting, weakness, weight loss, diarrhea, melena, and dehydration is often found. Polyuria, polydipsia, and trembling are sometimes present.

♥ In more severe cases, weakness, dehydration, weak pulses, collapse, and bradycardia are present, consistent with an Addisonian crisis.

✔ Lethargy is common as are weight loss, anorexia and weakness.

✔ The course can be waxing and waning.

✔ Clinical signs often respond to basic supportive care so that there may be a delay in establishing a definitive diagnosis.

Renal

✔ Without aldosterone, less potassium is excreted and sodium is lost excessively. Along with sodium, water is lost leading to polyuria and polydipsia. Hypotension and hypovolemia occur and this results in decreased renal perfusion.

♥ Decreased renal perfusion results in prerenal azotemia. With continued hypoperfusion true renal failure can occur.

✔ Urine specific gravity is low; this may be a result of renal medullary washout.

Cardiovascular

✔ The predominant cardiac manifestations of hypoadrenocorticism are related to hyperkalemia and hypovolemia because of hyponatremia.

✔ Hypotension may also be partially a result of decreased vascular catecholamine receptors.

♥ A patient with hypoadrenocorticism is often presented hypotensive and in shock. Although the expected compensatory response would be tachycardia, bradycardia is often detected.

✔ The ECG can show changes consistent with hyperkalemia such as lack of visible P-waves and tall and spiked T-waves (Figure 6-1). Other abnormalities include bradycardia, prolonged QRS duration, heart block and ventricular premature beats.

Gastrointestinal

✔ Commonly, GI problems are a presenting complaint for hypoadrenocorticism.

✔ A great majority of dogs have vomiting and/or diarrhea.

✔ Hemorrhage into the GI tract can occur. This may be because glucocorticoids are needed to maintain mucosal integrity. Decreased perfusion would also predispose to development of GI ulcers.

✔ Significant GI hemorrhage can contribute to azotemia.

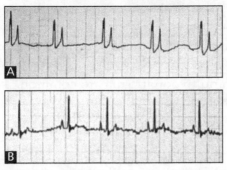

Figure 6-1 A. Electrocardiogram from a 4 yr, spayed female mixed breed dog with hypoadrenocorticism and a serum potassium of 7.1 mEq/L. Bradycardia (heart rate 68 bpm), lack of visible P-waves, and increased amplitude of the T-waves is typical of hyperkalemia. **B**. Electrocardiogram from the same dog as Figure 6-1A after 8 hours of treatment consisting of intravenous fluids and hydrocortisone. Note the increase in heart rate, reappearance of normal P-waves, and normal amplitude of the T-waves.

Uncommon Clinical Signs

Megaesophagus

✓ This is a relatively rare manifestation of hypoadrenocorticism. It is more significant in dogs with atypical disease where it can be a major presenting complaint and a potential source of severe complications such as aspiration pneumonia.

Neurologic

✓ Occasionally hypoglycemia can be one of the major presenting problems noted. Weakness and trembling can occur; in more severe cases seizures are noted.

Routine Laboratory Tests

✓ A variety of abnormalities can be detected in hypoadrenocorticism, whereby none are specific enough to allow a definitive diagnosis.

✓ A non-regenerative, normochromic, normocytic anemia is often present.

✓ The anemia can result from GI hemorrhage or chronic disease and glucocorticoid deficiency.

✓ Initially anemia can be masked by dehydration.

✓ Lymphocytosis and eosinophilia can occur.

♥ The lack of a stress leukogram in a very ill patient should raise suspicion of hypoadrenocortism.

✓ Hypoalbuminemia is common. This may be from increased GI blood loss, protein losing enteropathy or decreased synthesis.

♥ Hyperkalemia and hyponatremia are common. These can occur with other diseases such as renal failure, chylous effusions, and GI disease (especially whipworm associated). The ratio of sodium to potassium is important; a value less then 27:1 is suspicious.

✓ Azotemia is common (>85% of cases) and reflects poor kidney perfusion and impairment of renal concentrating ability. In most instances urine will be poorly concentrated, even with dehydration.

✓ Liver enzyme elevations have occasionally been documented; this could be the result of poor perfusion.

✓ Hypercalcemia is seen in about 30% of cases and is usually mild.

✓ Hypoglycemia is a reflection of glucocorticoid deficiency. Glucocorticoids act to increase hepatic glycogen and glucose production. It can be severe enough to cause clinical signs such as trembling, agitation, and seizures.

Diagnostic Imaging

✓ Diagnostic imaging rarely is of benefit in this disease since findings are non-specific.

✓ Radiographic changes noted include microcardia, diminished size of the caudal vena cava, small liver, and decreased size of the cranial lobar pulmonary artery.

✓ Megaesophagus, though rare, would also be a potential radiographic finding.

✓ Ultrasonography can reveal diminished size of the adrenal glands, especially in regard to width, though there is overlap between normal and Addisonian dogs.

Specific Tests for Diagnosis

♥ Hypoadrenocorticism is diagnosed by the lack of response to an ACTH stimulation test. Basal cortisol concentrations are usually low, however only dynamic testing with ACTH will allow a definitive diagnosis.

💣※ Use of corticosteroids other than dexamethasone (prednisone, prednisolone, hydrocortisone) prior to testing can interfere with cortisol results. If this has occurred switch to dexamethasone and wait 24 hours before testing.

✓ Obtain blood sample for measurement of cortisol before and 1 hour after administration of synthetic ACTH at 5µg /kg or 0.25 mg (1 vial) IV or IM.

✓ Natural ACTH (ACTH Gel) is given at a dose of 2.2 IU/kg IM. A serum sample is collected prior to and 2 hours after injection to assay cortisol concentration. Bioactivity of ACTH gel preparations is variable, so synthetic ACTH is recommended for testing.

✓ Interpretation of an ACTH Stimulation test: Hypoadrenocorticism is diagnosed when post-ACTH cortisol concentration is less than 2 µg/dL, values less than 4 µg/dl are highly suspicious.

Secondary Tests

✓ In cases where atypical hypoadrenocorticism is diagnosed, endogenous ACTH concentration can be determined. If elevated, the hypoadrenocorticism is primary (adrenal destruction), if low it is secondary (decreased ACTH production).

Treatment Recommendations

Objectives

✓ When dogs are presented in an Addisonian crisis, it is essential that appropriate interventions be instituted rapidly. In severe cases the animals are in shock and can easily go on to develop organ failure, especially renal failure.

✓ Long-term therapy focuses on maintaining a normal sodium to potassium ratio and preventing problems stemming from glucocorticoid deficiency such as weakness, GI signs, and inability to deal with stress.

Initial Treatment of the Addisonian Crisis

Fluids

♥ Fluid therapy is needed to reestablish perfusion and treat the hypovolemia. Crystalloid fluids such as 0.9% NaCl (preferred) or LRS are appropriate for this.

♥ Shock doses (40-80 ml/kg/hour) of fluids are used initially until the cardiovascular condition of the patient stabilizes. This will also help to decrease elevated potassium values.

♠ Rapid resolution of severe hyponatremia rarely causes severe CNS signs due to the rapid increase in osmolality following fluid therapy (see complications below).

Hyperkalemia

♥ Fluid therapy will reduce potassium by dilution and by increasing renal excretion and usually lowers potassium adequately without additional specific treatment.

♥ If hyperkalemia is severe, sodium bicarbonate (1-2 mEq/kg very slowly IV) can be used in addition to fluid therapy.

♥ Severe hyperkalemia can also be treated by intravenous administration of glucose and insulin (0.5 units/kg regular insulin with 3 g of glucose/unit of insulin; one-half of the glucose should be given as a bolus while the remainder should be administered over 6 hours in the intravenous fluids). Blood glucose should be monitored hourly during this treatment.

♥ Dextrose supplementation can also help to decrease potassium values as well as helping to combat hypoglycemia if symptomatic.

♥ Calcium can be given intravenously in severe cases of hyper-kalemia (calcium gluconate 10% solution; 0.5-1 ml/kg IV over 10 minutes), though many dogs with hypoadrenocorticism already have elevated calcium values.

Glucocorticoid Deficiency

♥ Glucocorticoid administration is generally advisable during initial therapy; dexamethasone is ideally suited for this since it will not interfere with the ACTH stimulation test. Initial dosage is 0.1-0.4 mg/kg IV.

✓ After the ACTH response test is completed, other corticosteroids can be administered.

♥ Hydrocortisone is the ideal replacement glucocorticoid because of its combination of mineralocorticoid and glucocorticoid activities. Administration of hydrocortisone sodium succinate at 0.3 mg/kg/h IV constant rate infusion or 2 mg/kg IV q 6 h.

✓ Other preparations such as prednisolone sodium succinate (1-2 mg/kg) can be used as well but cross-react when trying to measure cortisol concentrations as will hydrocortisone.

Mineralocorticoid Deficiency

✓ Mineralocorticoid deficiency does not have to be corrected on an emergency basis since many of the abnormalities resulting from it are corrected by fluid therapy. There is however little harm in administering short-acting mineralocorticoid supplements to an animal with normal adrenal function, so, therapy is instituted as soon as feasible in many cases.

✓ Fludrocortisone acetate at 0.01 mg/kg q 12 h orally is an effective therapy. Administration should be delayed until any vomiting is controlled.

✓ Desoxycorticosterone pivalate (DOCP, 2.2 mg/kgIM or SQ) is a long acting mineralocorticoid. While it can be used in dogs that are vomiting, it's use should be delayed until a definitive diagnosis of hypoadrenocorticism has been established.

✓ The chronic management of this disease requires frequent monitoring and changes in the amount and type of medications needed.

Complications

✓ Supportive care and administration of glucocorticoids and mineralocorticoids will usually result in resolution of all clinical abnormalities.

💣 Myelinolysis can occur with depression, weakness, ataxia, and spastic quadraparesis because of too rapid correction of hyponatremia by fluid therapy. As a result of the development of chronic hyponatremia, the brain compensates by decreasing intracellular osmolality (changes in inorganic ions and amino acids, so called idiogenic osmoles). The amino acids can only translocate slowly so it is possible for a significant diffusion gradient to develop. With correction of hyponatremia the cells dehydrate. This has been documented infrequently and occurs 1 to 4 days after treatment is initiated.

♥ The recommendation is to correct hyponatremia <12 mEq/L/day.

Long-Term Management of Hypoadrenocorticism

Mineralocorticoids

♥ Not required in dogs with atypical hypoadrenocorticism.

Fludrocortisone Acetate

✓ There is some glucocorticoid activity present so that it often is not necessary to supplement with glucocorticoids. This does, however, mean that polyuria and signs of hyperadrenocorticism can develop.

✓ With prolonged fludrocortisone therapy, the dose administered often needs to be increased to maintain good control.

✓ In large dogs with increasing dosages cost can become an important factor limiting the use of this medication.

✓ Electrolytes are checked every 7 to 14 days and dosages are adjusted until electrolytes normalize.

Desoxycorticosterone Pivalate

✓ Injections of DOCP (1-3 mg/kg IM or SQ) are given every 25 days. Initial dosage is 2.2 mg/kg and serum electrolytes are monitored at 12 and 25 days after the injection. If electrolytes are abnormal (hyponatremia, hyperkalemia) at 12 days, dosage is increased by 5 to 10%. If normal at 12, but abnormal at 25 days the dosing frequency may need to be decreased. If electrolytes are normal at 25 days repeatedly it may be possible to increase the interval between injections.

✓ It is the drug of choice when dogs become resistant to fludrocortisone or have PU/PD on fludrocortisone.

✓ Since DOCP has little if any glucocorticoid activity, it is necessary to supplement with physiologic doses of corticosteroids in most dogs.

✓ Treatment can be administered by owners after the appropriate dosage is established.

Glucocorticoids

✓ Prednisone or prednisolone are recommended for routine use.

✓ With fludrocortisone routine glucocorticoid replacement therapy is often not necessary after initial control of the hypoadrenocorticism.

♥ If there is a high stress situation (surgery, illness, athletic competition, etc.) it is advisable to supplement with glucocorticoids (prednisone 0.5 mg/kg/day).

✔ Most dogs on DOCP will need glucocorticoid supplementation (prednisone 0.2 mg/kg/day).

✔ The lowest dose of prednisone that controls clinical signs should be administered to reduce the likelihood of iatrogenic hyperadrenocorticism.

Salt Supplementation

✔ Generally this is not needed; mineralocorticoid therapy should be adjusted to control hyponatremia.

✔ Administration of NaCl (0.1 g/kg/day orally) may be useful if hyponatremia persists in dogs receiving fludrocortisone.

Monitoring

✔ Sodium and potassium values should be monitored regularly. Once stable on medications, every 3 to 6 months is sufficient.

✔ Patients with atypical hypoadrenocorticism should be monitored periodically for progression to mineralocorticoid deficiency, especially if an endogenous ACTH concentration was not measured initially to differentiate between primary and secondary hypoadrenocorticism.

Prognosis

Prognosis is generally good for treatment of this disease. Median survival with therapy is close to 5 years. Frequent monitoring is needed in these patients and the medications can be costly.

Feline Hypoadrenocorticism

✔ Clinical signs are similar to those seen in dogs.

✔ Very rare disease.

✔ Results from destruction of the adrenal cortex.

Diagnosis

♥ ACTH stimulation testing is also the basis for the diagnosis of hypoadrenocorticism in cats.

✔ The expected results are similar to dogs with post ACTH concentrations typically <1.5 ug/dL.

✔ If synthetic ACTH is used, 0.125 mg (half a vial) is given IM, blood is drawn 30 and 60 minutes later.

✓ With ACTH gel, 2.2 U/kg are given IM and blood is sampled at 60 and 120 minutes.

Treatment

✓ Treatment is similar to dogs, including aggressive fluid therapy, glucocorticoids and mineralocorticoids once a diagnosis is confirmed.

✓ Response to therapy may be delayed for several days, but most cats recover fully.

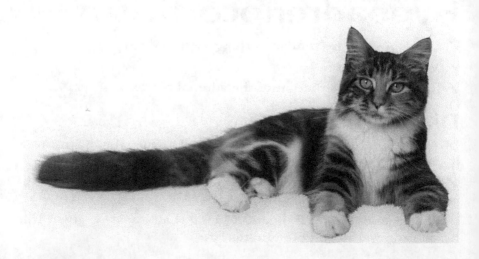

Section 7

Hyperaldosteronism

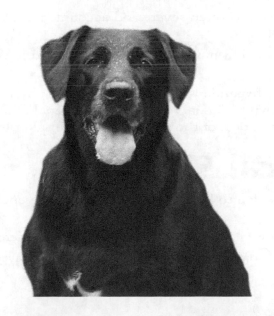

♥ **Problems**

Hypertension

Hypokalemia

Metabolic alkalosis

Hypernatremia

Blindness

Retinal hemorrhage

Weakness

Polyuria

Polydipsia

Weight loss

Heart murmur

Adrenal gland mass

Overview

✓ Primary hyperaldosteronism is caused by excessive secretion of aldosterone by an adrenocortical tumor or possibly by idiopathic bilateral adrenal gland hyperplasia.

♥ Excessive aldosterone results in retention of sodium and increased renal excretion of potassium and hydrogen ions, resulting in hypokalemia and metabolic alkalosis.

♥ Hypertension is often severe and accounts for many of the clinical signs.

✓ Rare disease, but more commonly recognized in the cat than in the dog.

✓ Secondary hyperaldosteronism is a normal physiologic response to hypovolemia, heart failure, or renal failure that results in activation of the renin-angiotensin-aldosterone system.

Clinical Signs

♥ Weakness, due to hypokalemia, is usually present, and may be episodic.

✓ Ventral cervical flexion may also be seen with severe hypokalemia.

✓ Myalgia is sometimes present, possibly due to hypokalemic myopathy.

♥ Polyuria and polydipsia are common, probably secondary to hypokalemia.

✓ A wide variety of CNS signs are possible due to brain hemorrhage secondary to hypertension.

♥ Retinal hemorrhage and subretinal effusion due to hypertensive retinopathy can cause blindness.

✓ Heart murmur secondary to cardiac changes induced by hypertension is common.

✓ An adrenal mass is palpable if sufficiently large.

⌐ Blood pressure is nearly always elevated.

Routine Laboratory Tests

⌐ Hypokalemia is the hallmark of hyperaldosteronism.

✓ Hypernatremia is less frequently present.

♥ Metabolic alkalosis is usually found, and may be suggested by finding an elevated total CO_2.

✓ Elevated creatine kinase activity secondary to hypokalemic polymyopathy.

✓ Urine specific gravity is typically <1.030 and is frequently nearly isosthenuric.

✓ Azotemia may be present secondary to pre-existing renal disease, hypertension-induced renal disease, or hypokalemic nephropathy.

Diagnostic Imaging

✓ Abdominal radiographs may show a mass cranial to either kidney consistent with an adrenal tumor.

♥ Abdominal ultrasound should reveal a mass involving one of the adrenal glands.

✓ Bilateral adrenomegaly may be present in rare cases of idiopathic hyperaldosteronism because of adrenal gland hyperplasia.

Specific Tests for Diagnosis

✓ Serum aldosterone concentration is elevated, usually markedly in primary hyperaldosteronism.

✓ Serum aldosterone concentration should be measured prior to fluid therapy or administration of diuretics or antihypertensive medications.

✓ Plasma renin activity must be measured concurrently to differentiate primary and secondary hyperaldosteronism.

✎ A diagnosis of primary hyperaldosteronism is made by finding an elevated serum aldosterone concentration with a concurrent low plasma renin activity.

✓ Secondary hyperaldosteronism is diagnosed when both serum aldosterone and plasma renin activity are elevated.

✓ A deoxycorticosterone-secreting tumor has been described in one dog; it had low serum aldosterone and plasma renin activity with elevated serum deoxycorticosterone.

Treatment Recommendations

✓ Definitive treatment is accomplished by removal of the adrenal gland tumor.

✓ Management of the hypertension and hypokalemia is recommended prior to surgery.

✓ Spironolactone is an aldosterone receptor antagonist that may be effective in increasing plasma potassium concentrations and decreasing the hypertensive effects of aldosterone.

✓ Low sodium diet can decrease renal potassium loss.

✓ Oral potassium supplementation should be provided as indicated.

✓ Specific treatment for hypertension should be undertaken if spironolactone administration does not decrease the blood pressure substantially.

✓ Amlodipine (0.625 mg QD) in cats and enalapril (0.5 mg/kg QD) in dogs are recommended for initial management of hypertension.

✓ It is difficult to reduce the blood pressure into the normal range in cats with primary hyperaldosteronism.

Prognosis

✓ The prognosis is good for animals in which the adrenal tumor is successfully removed at surgery.

✓ Retinal disease and blindness are often irreversible.

✓ Hypertension generally resolves after surgery.

✓ Hypertension is difficult to successfully manage without surgery.

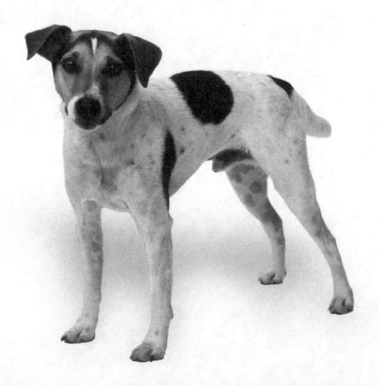

Section 8
Pheochromocytoma

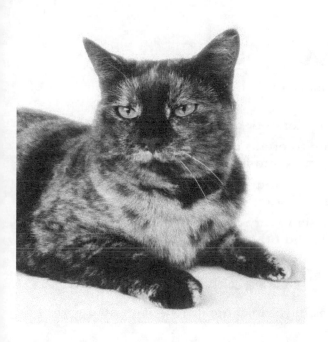

♥ Problems

Weakness

Anorexia

Collapse

Polyuria and polydipsia

Vomiting

Ascites or hemoabdomen

Abdominal mass

Tachyarrhythmia

Panting or dyspnea

Cough

Hypertension

Pale mucous membranes

Overview

✓ Pheochromocytoma is a rare tumor of the chromaffin cells of the adrenal medulla.

✓ Tumors may be functional or nonfunctional.

♥ Clinical signs relate to production of catecholamines or to the local effects of tumor mass and invasion of surrounding structures.

♥ Local tumor invasion is found in about 50% of cases and regional lymph node or distant metastasis is present in 15-25%.

♥ Concurrent neoplasia is very common (up to 50%), including adrenocortical tumors and other endocrine tumors.

Clinical Signs

✓ About 50% of dogs have no clinical signs associated with the pheochromocytoma.

♥ Nonspecific clinical signs occur most commonly, including weight loss, weakness, and anorexia.

✓ PU/PD is present in about 1/4 of cases.

✓ Collapse due to hypertensive crisis or intra-abdominal bleeding is relatively common.

✓ Pale mucous membranes occur in 1/3 of cases.

✓ Tachypnea, panting, and dyspnea are relatively common.

✓ Tachyarrhythmias including ventricular premature contractions are present in many dogs.

✓ Abdominal distension due to hemorrhage or ascites and palpable abdominal masses occur in about 15% of cases.

✓ Occasionally, seizures and paresis can occur.

✓ Signs due to a space occupying effect or vascular invasion are found in about 10%.

✓ Systemic arterial hypertension is common, but the true incidence is unknown and sometimes it may be associated with concurrent disorders rather than the pheochromocytoma.

Routine Laboratory Tests

✓ Nonspecific changes are common on the CBC, including leukocytosis, thrombocytopenia, and thrombocytosis.

✓ Elevations of liver enzyme activity are common.

✓ Hypoalbuminemia can be present and may be severe.

✓ Hypercholesterolemia is sometimes identified.

✓ Renal dysfunction appears to be common and is associated with elevated BUN, creatinine, and phosphorus and proteinuria.

Diagnostic Imaging

☝ Abdominal radiographs and ultrasonography are extremely valuable tools in the diagnosis of pheochromocytoma since clinical signs and clinicopathologic findings are generally nonspecific. Finding an adrenal mass may be the first indication that a pheochromocytoma is causing the clinical abnormalities.

♥ Abdominal ultrasound identifies the primary tumor and can aid in identification of metastasis.

♥ Careful evaluation of surrounding structures including the caudal vena cava, renal vasculature, and kidneys is necessary since invasion of these structures is common and is a major factor determining the success of surgical treatment.

✓ Venography of the caudal vena cava is probably the most sensitive technique for preoperative identification of invasion of the vena cava.

✓ CT of the abdomen is also useful for staging the tumor prior to surgery.

✓ Thoracic radiographs are indicated in all cases since pulmonary metastasis occurs.

Specific Tests for Diagnosis

♥ Preoperative confirmation of a pheochromocytoma is difficult. This neoplasm must be differentiated from adrenocortical tumors causing hyperadrenocorticism or hyperaldosteronism, both of which can cause hypertension.

✔ Measurement of plasma or urinary catecholamines or catecholamines metabolites is impractical in most veterinary practices.

✔ Pharmacological testing, such as measurement of blood pressure after phentoalmine administration is an unreliable and potentially dangerous method of diagnosis.

✔ Scintigraphy with metaiodobenzylguanidine (MIBG) can identify pheochromocytomas, but its use is limited by availability.

♥ Fine-needle aspirate of the adrenal mass may be an effective method of diagnosis and is practical in dogs and cats.

Treatment Recommendations

♥ Surgical adrenalectomy is the only definitive treatment.

✔ Management of hypertension can be accomplished prior to surgery or in nonsurgical cases by administration of phenoxybenzamine or prazosin.

✔ Because of the highly invasive nature of pheochromocytoma and the risk of catecholamines release caused by tumor manipulation during surgery, referral to an experienced specialist is suggested.

Prognosis

✔ Variable, depending on tumor characteristics, size, invasiveness, and functional aspects.

✔ Successful surgical removal of the tumor should result in long-term survival.

✔ Some dogs survive many months to years despite the presence of an invasive neoplasm.

Section 9

Diabetes Mellitus

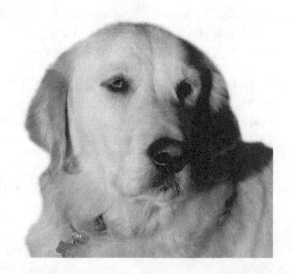

♥ **Problems**

Polyuria

Polydipsia

Polyphagia

Weight loss

Anorexia

Peripheral neuropathy

Ataxia

Cataracts

Urinary tract infection

Hepatomegaly

Hyperglycemia

Glycosuria

Hypercholesterolemia

Hyperlipidemia

Overview

✔ Diabetes mellitus is a common disease that results from a relative lack of insulin.

✔ Type I diabetes mellitus is an absolute insulin deficiency caused by destruction of beta-islet cells in the pancreas and is common in the dog.

✔ Type II diabetes mellitus appears to be common in the cat and is caused by insulin resistance combined with inadequate insulin secretion (type II diabetes mellitus). Obesity, age, and male gender are known risk factors for development of diabetes in cats. There is currently no noninvasive test to differentiate type I and type II diabetes mellitus in cats.

✔ Hyperadrenocorticism, acromegaly, and high progesterone states or administration of glucocorticoids or progestins can result in insulin resistance sufficient to cause diabetes mellitus in predisposed dogs and cats.

Transient Diabetes Mellitus in Cats

♥ Some cats have transient diabetes mellitus and no longer require insulin or oral hypoglycemic treatment. Recurrent hypoglycemia despite reduction of insulin dose typically occurs. Resolution of the diabetes is likely to occur within the first 2-4 months after diagnosis. Treatment for diabetes can be discontinued in these cases, but some cats will have a recurrence of diabetes months to years later.

Clinical Signs

⌫ Some combination of polyuria, polydipsia, polyphagia or inappetence, and weight loss are the most common clinical signs in dogs and cats with diabetes mellitus.

✓ Complications of diabetes mellitus are sometimes the primary complaint for presentation of some animals.

♥ Cats with peripheral neuropathy have hind limb weakness, a plantigrade stance, and hyporeflexia (Figure 9-1).

♥ Cataracts occur in at least 75% of diabetic dogs, with blindness resulting in many affected patients, while they are rare in cats with diabetes mellitus.

♥ Concurrent illness, particularly urinary tract infection, pancreatitis, and hyperadrenocorticism can also account for clinical findings in some diabetic dogs and cats.

♥ Physical examination may reveal hepatomegaly, muscle wasting, poor hair coat, dehydration, and renomegaly (cats) in addition to cataracts and signs of peripheral neuropathy.

✓ Systemic arterial hypertension may be present.

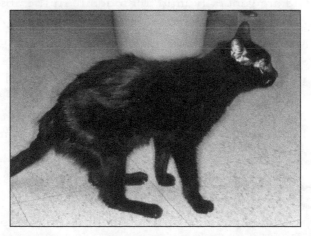

Figure 9-1 Peripheral neuropathy in a cat with diabetes mellitus. Note the typical plantigrade stance.

Routine Laboratory Tests

☞ The diagnosis of diabetes mellitus is made by demonstrating persistent, fasting hyperglycemia (>200-250 mg/dl in the dog; >300-350 mg/dl in the cat) and glycosuria in a patient with appropriate clinical signs.

♥ Stress hyperglycemia can result in elevation of blood glucose up to about 250 mg/dl in dogs and 400 mg/dl in cats.

✓ Glycosuria is present in virtually all animals with clinical signs of diabetes mellitus.

✓ Ketones present in large amounts in urine generally indicate ketoacidosis, but small amounts of ketones are often present in otherwise healthy diabetic dogs and less frequently cats.

✓ Proteinuria may indicate urinary tract infection or can be present due to diabetic nephropathy and subsequent glomerulosclerosis.

♥ Urinary tract infections occur in 20-40% of dogs and about 15% of cats with diabetes mellitus. Pyuria may or may not be present in these cases.

♥ Urine culture is indicated in all dogs and cats with newly diagnosed diabetes mellitus.

✓ Complete blood count may reveal hemoconcentration secondary to mild dehydration and occasionally leukocytosis in dogs and cats with uncomplicated diabetes mellitus.

✓ Elevated serum alkaline phosphatase (ALP) and alanine aminotransferase (ALT) activities are present in over 50% of diabetics, and are generally mild to moderate in the absence of concurrent disease.

✓ Hypercholesterolemia and hypertriglyceridemia are consistent findings.

✓ Mild hypoalbuminemia possibly secondary to renal loss and catabolism occurs in some diabetic dogs

✓ Other abnormalities sometimes found include electrolyte abnormalities, azotemia, hyperproteinemia, and hyperbilirubinemia, particularly in cats.

Diagnostic Imaging

✓ Dogs with uncomplicated diabetes mellitus do not routinely require diagnostic imaging.

✓ Emphysematous cystitis (Figure 9-2), cystic calculi, and pyelonephritis may be found in animals with urinary tract infections.

✓ Abdominal ultrasound can also be useful in evaluating diabetics that are difficult to control, with pancreatitis, pancreatic neoplasia, hepatic disease, adrenomegaly, and renal abnormalities occurring most often.

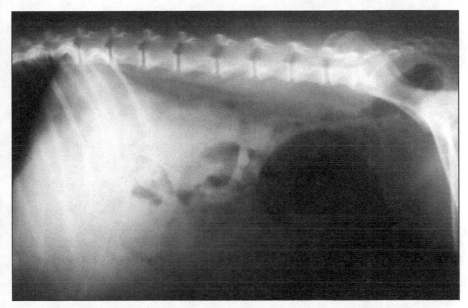

Figure 9-2 Emphysematous cystitis in a dog with diabetes mellitus and a urinary tract infection.

Specific Tests for Diagnosis

♥ Typical clinical findings combined with hyperglycemia and glycosuria are sufficient for diagnosis of diabetes mellitus in almost all cases.

✓ Stress hyperglycemia in cats can usually be differentiated from diabetes by repeating the blood glucose after hospitalizing the cat for a few hours.

Treatment Recommendations

☞ Goals of treatment of diabetes mellitus are to:

Eliminate clinical signs

Prevent complications of diabetes mellitus such as cataracts and diabetic neuropathy

Avoid complications of treatment such as hypoglycemia

Maintain acceptable blood glucose concentrations

Resolve the diabetes in cats

✋ Strict control of blood glucose should be attempted in:

Dogs that have not developed cataracts

Cats with peripheral neuropathy

Animals prone to develop diabetic ketoacidosis

♥ The risk of hypoglycemia increases with attempts at strict regulation of blood glucose.

Exercise

✓ Enhanced control of diabetes can be accomplished by moderate, consistent exercise.

✋ Strenuous exercise such as hunting will be associated with a substantial reduction in insulin requirements, so the dose of insulin should be reduced by at least 50% the day exercise is planned and a glucose source should be readily available in case of symptomatic hypoglycemia.

Diet

♥ Dogs should be fed a restricted fat, moderate protein diet high in complex carbohydrates that contains increased amounts of dietary fiber.

✓ The main effect of fiber is to slow the absorption of glucose from the small intestine, thus reducing the degree of postprandial hyperglycemia to a modest degree.

✋ Cats fed a low carbohydrate, high protein (approximately 50% protein) diet, are more likely to have resolution of their diabetes than cats fed a high carbohydrate, high fiber diet. Many cats treated with insulin and a low carbohydrate diet have resolution of their diabetes mellitus.

✓ Obese animals should be fed a dietary regimen that results in weight loss, since obesity induces insulin resistance.

✓ Underweight animals should be fed a high quality food that has a high caloric density until normal body condition is reached.

✓ Avoid diets such as semi-moist food that contain high quantities of simple carbohydrates.

♥ Animals should be fed at the time of insulin administration when treated twice per day or at the time of feeding and if possible 1-2 hours prior to the peak insulin effect when treated once per day.

✓ Cats and dogs that are not trained to eat a full meal at a specific time should have dry food available at all times.

Insulin Treatment

✓ Insulin administration is the mainstay of treatment of diabetes mellitus in the dog and cat.

✓ Insulins used for routine management of uncomplicated diabetes mellitus are complexed with substances such as protamine and zinc to delay their absorption after subcutaneous administration (Table 9-1).

Table 9-1
Insulins used for Management of Diabetes Mellitus

Insulin Type	Onset of Action	Duration of Action Dog	Cat	Comments
Regular	Immediate IV; 10-30 minutes IM, SQ	1-4 hr 3-8 hr	1-4 hr 3-8 hr	Use for ketoacidosis, rarely combined with other insulins
NPH	.5-3 hr	4-24 hr	4-12 hr	Often < 10 hr duration in cats
Lente	< 1 hr	8-24 hr	6-24 hr	Mixture of regular and ultralente; has 2 different peak effect times; pork product (Vetsulin®) approved for dogs and cats
Ultralente	2-8 hr	8-28 hr	8-24 hr	Sometimes poorly absorbed in cat
PZI	1-4 hr	6-28 hr	6-24 hr	Beef/pork product marketed for use in cats; use of compounded product is not recommended
Insulin Lispro	Rapid	Unknown in dog and cat		Short acting insulin analog similar to regular insulin
Glargine insulin	1-4 hr	Unknown	10-16 hr	Long-acting insulin analog

♥ The duration of action varies widely in individual patients, so treatment must be adjusted according to the response of each patient.

♥ The insulins preferred by the authors are lente and PZI in cats and lente and NPH in the dog.

✓ Insulin glargine has been used successfully in cats and may result in less fluctuation of blood glucose than other insulins when administered every 12 hours.

♥ Dogs can be successfully managed with NPH insulin, but its duration of action is often too short for optimal treatment of cats.

✓ Ultralente insulin is effective in cats, but 15-20% will not absorb ultralente insulin adequately and require very high doses.

✓ Ultralente or PZI insulin is preferred if once daily insulin treatment is a goal for cat owners.

✓ Because of the periodic discontinuation of some insulin of animal and human origin, we recommend the use of products approved for veterinary use, human recombinant insulin, or insulin analogs for use in all newly diagnosed diabetics. Only products approved for veterinary use have been thoroughly evaluated in clinical trials of dogs and cats.

✓ When using a low dose of insulin (<2 u) products with a concentration of 40 u/ml (PZI, Porcine lente insulin for veterinary use) are recommended.

💣 The proper insulin syringe should be used with each product. Failure to use a 40 u/ml syringe with veterinary insulins of this concentration may result in a substantial under dose. Use of a 40 u/ml syringe for 100 u/ml insulin will result in a potentially life-threatening insulin overdose.

✓ Syringes with 0.3 ml capacity can increase accuracy in administering small doses of insulin.

Monitoring Insulin Treatment

♥ The initial insulin dose is 0.5 units/kg in the dog and 0.5 units/kg or 1-3 units in the cat.

♥ Treatment can be initiated once or twice daily, but the majority of animals are best managed with twice daily insulin.

♥ Blood glucose concentration should be monitored 2-3 times 4-8 hours after the first insulin injection to ensure that hypoglycemia does not occur at this dose.

♥ The animal should then be released after the owner is counseled on insulin handling, injection technique, and monitoring for clinical signs of inadequate control of diabetes and hypoglycemia.

💣 When feeding a low carbohydrate, high protein food to a cat, insulin requirements may decrease rapidly after diet change, so cats must be monitored for carefully for signs of hypoglycemia. Complete glucose curves should be evaluated weekly because the insulin dose usually needs to be decreased after 1-2 weeks of treatment. Resolution of diabetes usually occurs after 4-8 weeks of treatment with low carbohydrate diet and insulin, but may occur at a later time in some cats.

Initial Monitoring

✓ The patient returns one week after initiating treatment for evaluation.

♥ The morning of the initial evaluation, the owner should feed the pet at home as usual, but not administer the insulin until observed by the attending veterinarian or veterinary technician. This provides an opportunity to address any deficiencies in injection technique and to address any concerns of the owner regarding insulin administration.

⚷ Clinical response is a very important tool in monitoring the response to insulin treatment, and correlates well with other measures of response including blood glucose curves and serum fructosamine.

♥ The owner should be asked a series of questions regarding the presence of polyuria, polydipsia, polyphagia, lethargy, or weakness in addition to inquiries about any problems with administration of insulin. A short questionnaire is convenient for owners to fill out when they drop off their dog or cat for assessment (Appendix 1).

Glucose Curve

Protocol

⚷ The glucose curve should be performed by obtaining blood samples for measurement of glucose every 2 hours for 8-12 hours in animals treated twice per day; if possible additional samples should be obtained at 16 and 24 hours after insulin when administered once per day.

♥ Less frequent sampling may result in significant hypoglycemia being overlooked.

💣 It is inappropriate to obtain "spot checks" (single blood glucose measurements) at the time that the peak effect of insulin is expected because the peak effect is unpredictable from one injection to another and may change depending on the insulin dosage.

✓ The blood glucose should ideally be assayed using an in house chemistry analyzer or the plasma or serum separated within 30 minutes of collection and assayed at a reference laboratory.

✔ The hand held glucose meters generally underestimate the glucose concentration and are somewhat inaccurate because of this. With this in mind, these units can be used, but should be compared with a reference assay to get a "feeling" about how the measurements vary from the laboratory standard.

✔ Venipuncture can be avoided by using a lancet to obtain a droplet of blood from the pinna of a cat or dog, which can be used to measure the glucose in the appropriate glucometer.

✔ Home monitoring of blood glucose is a practical alternative to in-hospital monitoring. It avoids the stress of hospitalization and repeated venipuncture. A lancing device is used to puncture the skin on the inner surface of the pinna and the drop of capillary blood is applied to a hand held glucometer. Owners must be trained in the proper use of this technique.

Interpretation

✔ The most important pieces of information obtained from a blood glucose curve are the blood glucose concentration at its nadir and the duration of effect (Figure 9-3).

♥ The lowest concentration that the glucose reaches during a glucose curve is the nadir, and the ideal concentration is 100-150 mg/dl.

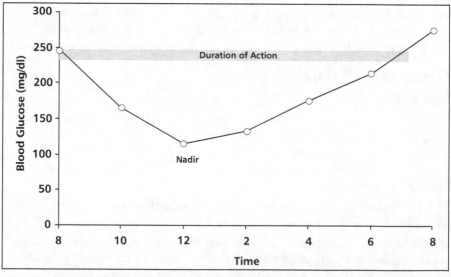

Figure 9-3 Sample glucose curve. Blood glucose curve in a dog receiving lente insulin twice per day at 8:00 a.m. and 8:00 p.m. The lowest blood glucose concentration, called the nadir, occurs at 12:00, 4 hours after the insulin injection. The duration of action is represented by the shaded area and is 11 hours, corresponding to the time the blood glucose is <250 mg/dl.

❤ The duration of effect is the time that the blood glucose remains below a target concentration, usually 200-250 mg/dl.

❤ The insulin dose usually needs to be increased if the nadir is >150 mg/dl. Blood glucose concentrations <80-100 mg/dl should prompt a reduction in the insulin dose.

✓ The magnitude of adjustment of insulin dose varies depending on the size of the patient, the degree of hyperglycemia or hypoglycemia, and current insulin dose. Adjustments generally range from 0.5 to 3 units per dose.

🖐 Stress can invalidate a glucose curve by inhibiting the action of insulin and elevating blood glucose (Figure 9-4). This problem mimics that of insulin resistance.

✓ There is considerable variation between glucose curves on sequential days, so the results of a glucose curve should be interpreted with other indicators of control (clinical signs, physical examination) in mind.

Insufficient Dose

✓ Underdosing will result in a nadir where the blood glucose is >150 mg/dl.

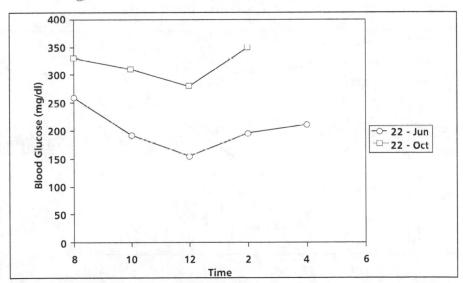

Figure 9-4 Effect of stress on blood glucose curve. Blood glucose curves on two different dates in a dog receiving twice daily NPH insulin at the same dose on each date. The dog had rapidly progressive cataracts and became blind shortly before the second blood glucose curve. The dog showed signs of severe stress during the glucose curve in October and had a poor response to insulin. The insulin dose was not changed and the dog's blood glucose curve improved after it became accustomed to its loss of sight.

✔ The duration of action may be difficult to determine because the nadir is not sufficiently low.

✔ Increase the dose of insulin by 0.5 to 1 unit per dose in cats, and 1 to 3 units per dose in the dog depending on size and adequacy of control.

Inadequate Duration of Action

✔ The duration of action is measured by the length of time that the blood glucose is < 250 mg/dl when the nadir blood glucose is between 100-150 mg/dl.

♥ The duration of action of insulin should be at least 20-24 hours in animals administered insulin once per day and 10-12 hours in those on twice daily treatment.

♥ If duration of action is too short on once daily treatment (Figure 9-5) but the glucose nadir is adequate, the insulin dose is reduced by approximately 25% and administered twice per day. If the nadir is inadequate, the insulin dose to be administered twice daily is reduced by <25%.

♥ If insulin is being administered twice per day and the duration is <10 hours, a longer acting insulin should be substituted. This occurs most frequently with NPH insulin in cats.

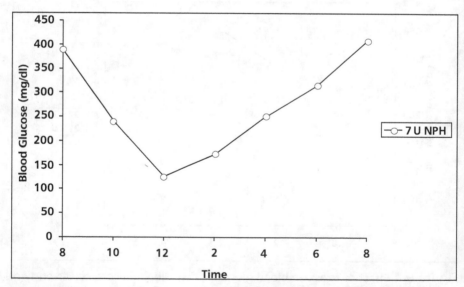

Figure 9-5 Short duration of action. Blood glucose curve in a dog receiving 7 units of NPH insulin twice per day at 8:00 a.m. and 8:00 p.m. The nadir occurs 4 hours after injection at a blood glucose concentration of 126 mg/dl. The blood glucose exceeds 250 mg/dl at 4 p.m., giving a duration of action of only 6-8 hours. The duration of action should be at least 10-11 hours for good control.

Insulin Overdose

✓ An overdose of insulin will result in a nadir on the blood glucose curve of <80 mg/dl.

✓ If mild hypoglycemia occurs, clinical signs may be absent and the blood glucose will gradually rise back into the normal range.

♥ A more substantial overdose will result in sustained hypoglycemia and possibly clinical signs or a rebound hyperglycemia.

💣 The subsequent insulin dose should be reduced by up to 50% and should not be administered until it is clear that the effect of the previously administered insulin has resolved (hyperglycemia is again present).

Insulin-induced Hyperglycemia (Somogyi Phenomenon)

✓ Insulin-induced hyperglycemia occurs after an overdose of insulin results in hypoglycemia followed by hyperglycemia. The counter-regulatory response to hypoglycemia involves release of glucagon, catecholamines, and cortisol that impair the effects of insulin and induce hyperglycemia.

♥ The glucose curve in Figure 9-6 depicts the initial hypoglycemia rapidly followed by marked hyperglycemia in a dog with insulin-induced hyperglycemia.

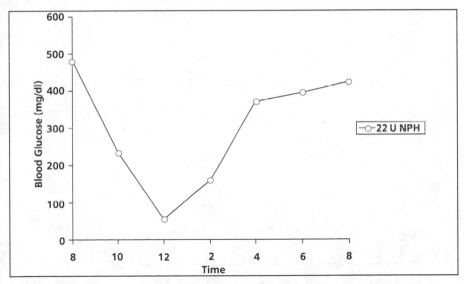

Figure 9-6 Insulin-induced hyperglycemia. Blood glucose curve of a miniature schnauzer receiving 22 U NPH insulin twice per day. The insulin dose was gradually increased over 4 months based on daily urine glucose monitoring. The nadir occurs 4 hours after injection at a blood glucose of 55 mg/dl. The rapid and marked rise in blood glucose is due to the counter-regulatory response induced by hypoglycemia.

✊ Because hyperglycemia is present for most of the day, clinical findings of polyuria, polydipsia, polyphagia, and glycosuria are identical to those when an insufficient dose of insulin is administered.

✔ Clinical signs of hypoglycemia are often absent or overlooked in this situation, making a complete glucose curve the only method that will reliably confirm insulin-induced hyperglycemia.

♥ A reduction in the insulin dose by 25% or more is indicated, and further dosage adjustment will be determined based on results of a glucose curve 5-7 days later.

Poor Insulin Response or Absorption

✔ Certain insulins appear to be poorly absorbed or have minimal activity in some cats.

✋ Ultralente insulin has minimal glucose-lowering effect in about 20% of cats; the occasional cat will have a similar response to lente insulin.

✔ Glucose curves in this instance show little or no decrease after insulin injection, even with doses exceeding 8-10 units twice per day (Figure 9-7).

♥ Administration of a standard dose (1-3 units) of a different insulin such as lente or PZI, will resolve the problem.

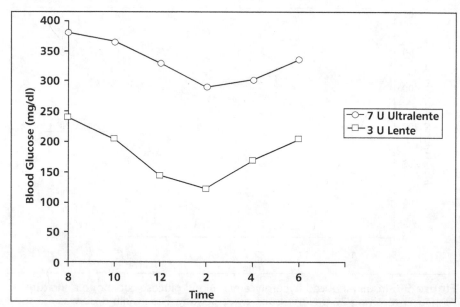

Figure 9-7 Poor absorption of ultralente insulin in a cat. Blood glucose curve in a cat receiving ultralente insulin twice daily. Note the minimal response to the ultralente insulin, mimicking insulin resistance. The insulin preparation was changed to lente and the cat responded as expected to a low dose.

Insulin Resistance

✓ Insulin resistance occurs when the response to a given dose of insulin is less than would be expected in an uncomplicated diabetic.

♥ An animal receiving >1.5-2.0 units/kg of insulin per dose without good control of blood glucose would be considered insulin resistant.

♥ The first objective in this situation is to rule out owner-generated problems including poor injection technique, inaccurate dosing, or inactive insulin.

✓ The potential medical causes of insulin resistance are numerous (Table 9-2), but most potential problems can be diagnosed with a thorough history, physical examination and routine laboratory testing including complete blood count, serum biochemical profile, urinalysis, urine culture, and serum T4 concentration.

Table 9-2
Causes of Insulin Resistance

Improper administration
Poor absorption of insulin
Infection

Endocrine disorders
    Hyperadrenocorticism
    Hyperthyroidism
    Hypothyroidism
    Acromegaly
    Diestrus
    Pheochromocytoma
    Glucagonoma

Drug administration
    Glucocorticoids
    Progestins

Obesity
Pancreatitis/exocrine pancreatic insufficiency
Neoplasia
Renal failure
Hepatic failure
Anti-insulin antibodies

✓ Administration of topical or systemic glucocorticoids and progestins can cause insulin resistance.

✓ Intact females are expected to develop insulin resistance during diestrus because of elevated progesterone, and should be spayed unless otherwise contraindicated.

🖐 Urinary tract infection is one of the most common causes so a urine culture should be performed in all cases of insulin resistant diabetes mellitus regardless of findings on urinalysis.

✓ Evaluation of adrenal function should be considered in all animals where clinical signs of hyperadrenocorticism are present or a cause of insulin resistance is not readily apparent.

✓ Hyperadrenocorticism and acromegaly can occur in cats without classical signs of these disorders. Evaluation of adrenal function tests and measurement of insulin-like growth factor-1 (IGF-1) should be considered in cats with unexplained insulin-resistant diabetes mellitus.

✓ Imaging of the pituitary gland using CT or MRI may be necessary to demonstrate a pituitary tumor.

✓ Chronic pancreatitis and pancreatic neoplasia appear to be common in cats that either have insulin resistant diabetes or are difficult to control.

♥ Abdominal ultrasound examination is useful for identification of pyelonephritis, pancreatitis, adrenal neoplasia, chronic cystitis, and various neoplasms.

✓ Insulin resistance should resolve after resolution of the cause, although diabetes mellitus may persist (Figure 9-8).

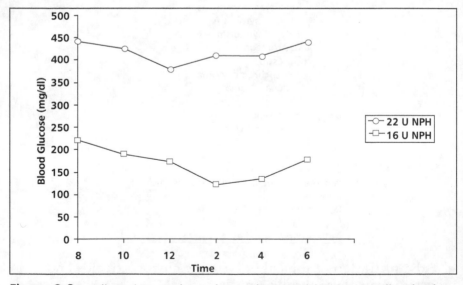

Figure 9-8 Insulin resistance due to hyperadrenocorticism in a Poodle. Blood glucoses curve of a dog with hyperadrenocorticism. Prior to treatment, the dog had poor glycemic control on 22 U NPH twice per day. After adequate treatment of the hyperadrenocorticism with mitotane, the insulin dose was reduced to 16 units and the diabetes was well controlled.

Alternatives to Blood Glucose Curves

Urine Glucose

✔ Urine glucose measurements are best used as an adjunct to other methods of monitoring, and are particularly useful in patients where a blood glucose curve may be invalid because of stress or when insulin requirements are expected to decrease.

🖐 Changes in insulin dose should not be made based solely on urine glucose concentrations since insulin-induced hyperglycemia can result in marked glycosuria despite an insulin overdose. The exception is when the urine glucose is negative during initial treatment of hyperadrenocorticism.

✔ The owner should keep a log of urine glucose measurements obtained at the same time of the day (first urination in the morning), several days per week, for the veterinarian to interpret.

✔ If measurements several days in a row have a marked elevation of urine glucose, the animal should be evaluated.

♥ Urine ketone measurement is useful in some animals that are prone to ketoacidosis or have concurrent illness.

Serum Fructosamine and Glycosylated Hemoglobin

✔ Prolonged hyperglycemia results in nonenzymatic glycosylation of proteins, including hemoglobin (glycosylated hemoglobin) and serum proteins (fructosamine).

✔ The concentration of glycosylated hemoglobin is a reflection of the blood glucose concentration over 3-4 months in the dog and about 2 months in the cat, while serum fructosamine is determined by the blood glucose over the previous 7-14 days.

✔ Concentrations of these compounds are not affected by transient, stress-induced hyperglycemia.

✔ A single blood sample is required.

✔ Fructosamine is more readily available; glycosylated hemoglobin must be measured by an assay method validated for use in the dog and cat.

✔ Elevated serum fructosamine is present in most, but not all diabetic dogs and cats, and can be used as an aid in the diagnosis of diabetes in selected cases.

✔ Well-controlled diabetic dogs and cats typically have mildly increased to normal fructosamine and glycosylated hemoglobin concentrations, while these proteins tend to remain elevated in poorly controlled patients.

There is considerable overlap in fructosamine and glycosylated hemoglobin concentrations in well controlled and poorly controlled diabetics, so measurement of these proteins alone is not sufficient to determine if control is adequate. Owner observations, physical examination and if available, glucose curves are important factors in assessing glycemic control.

Hypoglycemia cannot be diagnosed using these methods, so it is prudent to measure blood glucose at the time a sample is obtained for glycosylated protein.

✓ Fructosamine concentration is decreased by hypoproteinemia, hyperlipidemia, azotemia, and uncontrolled hyperthyroidism, while glycosylated hemoglobin is decreased by anemia.

Chronic Monitoring Recommendations

✓ Routine rechecks should be scheduled every 3-4 months for history, physical examination, and body weight.

♥ If the animal appears well controlled on the basis of these evaluations, no further testing or dosage adjustment is indicated.

✓ Fructosamine or glycosylated hemoglobin could be measured, but dosage adjustments should not be made based on an elevated glycosylated protein in an animal that is well controlled clinically.

♥ If there is indication that a diabetic dog or cat is not well controlled, appropriate testing such as a glucose curve and/or fructosamine should be evaluated.

✓ Urinalysis and urine culture should be considered prior to other diagnostic testing in poorly controlled animals.

Oral Hypoglycemic Agents

✓ Glipizide is an oral sulfonylurea drug that enhances release of insulin from pancreatic islet cells, so it is probably only effective in cats with type II diabetes mellitus. There is no indication for its use in dogs with diabetes mellitus.

✓ Good glycemic control is reached in 20-25% of cats treated with glipizide, while cats that do not respond require treatment with insulin after cessation of glipizide administration.

♥ In order to be a candidate for treatment with glipizide, a cat must be in normal to obese body condition, should not have suffered considerable recent weight loss, not be ketotic, and not have concurrent illness.

♥ Treatment protocol:

Administer glipizide at 2.5 mg PO BID with food for 2 weeks.

Perform a history, physical examination, 8-hour glucose curve, and urine ketones weekly until an adequate response is achieved.

Increase the dose to 5 mg PO BID if euglycemia is not reached in 2 weeks, continuing weekly evaluations.

Treatment is continued provided control of the diabetes is considered adequate based on clinical signs and blood glucose curves.

Discontinue treatment if no response is present after 4-8 weeks of treatment, clinical signs including weight loss worsen, ketonuria is detected, or if side effects of vomiting or icterus occur.

If hypoglycemia occurs, the dose should be gradually tapered and discontinued if hyperglycemia does not recur.

✓ Side effects include vomiting, icterus, and elevated liver enzymes.

✓ Side effects resolve after decreasing the dose of glipizide or discontinuing treatment.

Other Oral Treatments

✓ Metformin, vanadium, chromium, troglitizone, and acarbose have been evaluated in small numbers of dogs and/or cats. Their utility remains to be demonstrated.

Insulin Treatment and General Anesthesia

✓ The insulin dose should be decreased in animals undergoing anesthesia.

♥ If the blood glucose the morning of surgery is higher than 140 mg/dl, 1/2 the normal insulin dose is administered.

♥ If the blood glucose is <140 mg/dl, 1/4 of the normal dose should be given.

⚬ Monitoring the blood glucose during and after surgery is essential since blood glucose and thus insulin requirements may vary considerably during the post-operative period. Dextrose containing intravenous fluid solutions should be administered as necessary to prevent hypoglycemia.

✋ Hypoglycemia may occur 10 or more hours after the previous dose of insulin.

Complications of Diabetes Mellitus

Cataracts

♥ Cataracts develop in most diabetic dogs, and about 50% are blind within 2 years of diagnosis.

✔ Diabetic cataracts are rare in the cat.

♥ Good control of the diabetic state may slow progression or possibly prevent cataract formation, but cataracts can form and blindness may occur rapidly despite appropriate treatment in some cases.

✔ Cataract removal will restore vision in the majority of dogs undergoing this surgery.

✔ Retinal function must be evaluated prior to surgery to ensure that an unrelated retinal disease causing blindness is not present.

♥ Uveitis can occur in some cases. Topical treatment with a nonsteroidal anti-inflammatory such as suprofen or flurbiprofen 2-4 times per day is preferred over topical glucocorticoids. Topical 1% atropine is indicated when the eye is painful and the pupil is constricted. Systemic treatment consists of carprofen, etodolac or another NSAID if necessary.

Peripheral Neuropathy

✔ Peripheral neuropathy is seen primarily in cats; this complication is usually subclinical in the dog.

♥ Hind limb weakness resulting in a plantigrade stance is the typical presenting complaint in affected cats (see Figure 9-1).

✔ Hyporeflexia, muscle atrophy, and postural deficits are also present.

♥ Strict control of the blood glucose is necessary in cats with diabetic neuropathy and will result in resolution of clinical signs in most cases.

Hypoglycemia

♥ Clinical signs include weakness, ataxia, collapse, seizures, restlessness, pacing, vomiting, diarrhea, depression, and lethargy.

♥ If recognized before severe signs, feeding the animal a normal meal may be sufficient to resolve the immediate problem. If the animal refuses to eat or continues to have clinical signs, a concentrated sugar solution (corn syrup, pancake syrup, honey, etc.) should be fed.

♥ If the animal is unconscious, a sugar solution should be applied to the gingival and labial mucosa. The owner should be instructed to never place a finger or other object in the mouth of a seizuring dog because injury is likely. Oral administration in these circumstances could result in aspiration.

♥ Intravenous administration of 50% dextrose (1 ml/kg) followed by a constant rate infusion of 2.5-10% dextrose (typically 5% initially) is most appropriate for in hospital management. Further discussion on treatment of hypoglycemia can be found in Section 11.

♥ In animals with symptomatic hypoglycemia, insulin treatment should be discontinued until hyperglycemia is documented, then reinstituted at not more than 50% of the previous dose.

Other Complications

♥ Urinary tract infection is common and frequently occurs without clinical signs. Urine culture should be performed during initial diagnostic testing and periodically (probably every 6-12 months) during treatment.

✓ Other infections, including conjunctivitis, stomatitis, and dermatologic infections (including demodecosis) also appear to be more common in diabetics. Hypertension is present in some diabetics, and hypertensive retinopathy has been reported in cats with diabetes mellitus.

✓ Diabetic retinopathy independent of hypertension occurs in some diabetic dogs and is manifest by pinpoint retinal hemorrhages. It does not appear to cause significant vision loss in dogs or cats.

✓ Pancreatitis and pancreatic exocrine insufficiency are sometimes present in dogs with diabetes mellitus, possibly as a cause of the diabetes rather than a consequence of it.

✓ Diabetic ketoacidosis and nonketotic hyperosmolar syndrome are discussed in the following chapter.

Prognosis

✓ Mean survival in diabetic dogs and cats is about 1-2 years.

✓ With proper management and consideration of the goals of treatment (eliminate clinical signs, prevent complications of diabetes mellitus, avoid complications of treatment, and maintain euglycemia), long-term survival should be attained.

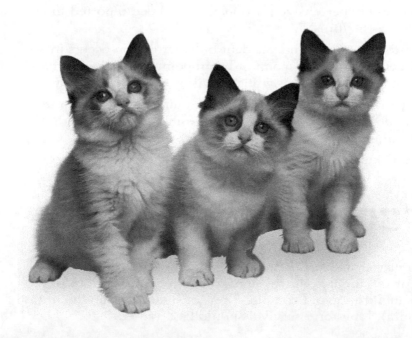

Section 10
Diabetic Ketoacidosis

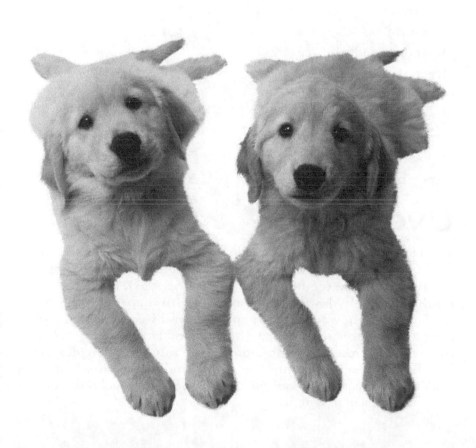

♥ Problems
Polyuria

Polydipsia

Polyphagia

Weight loss

Lethargy

Anorexia

Vomiting

Dehydration

Icterus

Hepatomegaly

Tachypnea

Abdominal pain

Hyperglycemia

Glycosuria

Ketonuria

Metabolic acidosis

Hypokalemia

Hyponatremia

Hypophosphatemia

Liver enzyme elevation

Hypocalcemia

Hypercholesterolemia

Overview

✓ Diabetic ketoacidosis is a life-threatening form of diabetes mellitus that results from a combination of factors including insulin resistance (counterregulatory hormones), fasting, a lack of insulin, and dehydration in an animal with diabetes mellitus. Insulin deficiency and insulin antagonism by counterregulatory hormones induces severe hyperglycemia and ketone body production that causes marked osmotic diuresis and results in dehydration and deficiencies in sodium, potassium, and phosphate. Metabolic acidosis also occurs and can have detrimental effects on the nervous and cardiovascular systems.

♥ Most animals with diabetic ketoacidosis have concurrent diseases that cause insulin resistance and anorexia. The prognosis is often related as much to the nature of the concurrent disease as to the ketoacidotic state.

Clinical Signs

♥ The classical signs of diabetes mellitus including polyuria, polydipsia, polyphagia, and weight loss are almost always present.

✋ A thorough history is important because owners may consider the more chronic signs unimportant in the presence of acute illness.

♥ Lethargy, anorexia, and vomiting are frequently present.

✓ Concurrent disease may cause a variety of historical abnormalities unrelated to the diabetic ketoacidosis.

✓ Many animals have not been previously diagnosed with diabetes mellitus.

♥ Physical examination findings include thin body condition, dehydration, depression, hepatomegaly, tachypnea, and an acetone odor to the breath.

♥ Clinical signs are often related to concurrent diseases including pancreatitis, infection, renal failure, neoplasia, cholangiohepatitis, hepatic lipidosis, and other disorders.

Routine Laboratory Tests

🔑 Hyperglycemia, glycosuria, and ketonuria are present in all cases.

✓ Metabolic acidosis is present as indicated by arterial blood gas or by total $CO_2 < 15$ mEq/L on serum chemistries.

✓ Inflammatory leukogram may be present.

✓ Serum biochemical abnormalities are similar to those of uncomplicated diabetes mellitus and can also include findings consistent with concurrent disease.

♥ Total body sodium, potassium, and phosphorus are usually depleted, but serum concentrations of these electrolytes are usually normal prior to treatment.

💣 Electrolytes should be monitored frequently during treatment because hypokalemia is very common, and hypophosphatemia and hyponatremia can occur.

♥ Urine culture should be performed in all cases because of a high incidence of urinary tract infection.

Diagnostic Imaging

✓ Abdominal radiographs and/or abdominal ultrasound are usually indicated in dogs and cats with diabetic ketoacidosis because of the high incidence of complications and concurrent disease such as pancreatitis, pyometra, prostatitis, urinary tract infection, and other diseases.

✓ Thoracic radiographs are necessary in some cases where pneumonia or metastatic neoplasia is suspected.

Specific Tests for Diagnosis

♥ Finding hyperglycemia, glycosuria, ketonuria, and metabolic acidosis combined with appropriate clinical signs is diagnostic of diabetic ketoacidosis.

Treatment Recommendations

♥ Diabetic dogs and cats with ketonuria that do not have clinical signs of illness other than those consistent with uncomplicated diabetes mellitus can be treated as a routine diabetic with an intermediate acting insulin alone. These animals do not have true ketoacidosis.

♥ More severe forms of diabetic ketoacidosis require a combination of intravenous fluids, insulin, electrolyte supplementation, and other supportive treatment.

Intravenous Fluid Therapy

⌖ Goals of IV fluid treatment are to replace volume deficits, improve tissue perfusion, replace electrolyte deficiencies, and to lower the blood glucose concentration.

♥ Normal saline is the fluid of choice, but other balanced electrolyte replacement solutions are acceptable.

✓ Administer fluids at a rate to replace fluid deficits over a 24 hour period, with 1/2 of the fluid deficit given over the first 4-6 hours.

💣 Urine production should be apparent within 2-4 hours of initiating IV fluid administration; lack of urine production may indicate acute, oliguric renal failure.

♥ Potassium supplementation should be instituted at the time IV fluid therapy is begun based on serum potassium concentration. If serum potassium concentration is not available, supplement fluids with 40 mEq/L KCl once adequate urine production has been documented (see below).

♥ Monitor serum potassium, sodium, and phosphorus every 8-12 hours.

✓ Adjust potassium supplementation and sodium administration (alter fluids to lactated Ringer's solution or 0.45% saline with 2.5% dextrose if hypernatremia occurs) as necessary.

Insulin Therapy

☛ The goals of insulin administration are to gradually decrease the blood glucose concentration without inducing hypoglycemia or marked hypokalemia, to halt ketone body formation, to increase ketone metabolism, and decrease lipolysis and protein catabolism.

Low-dose Intramuscular Insulin Treatment

✓ Initial dose of regular insulin is 0.2 U/kg IM.

✓ Subsequent hourly dose is 0.1 U/kg IM until the blood glucose ≤ 250 mg/dl.

✓ The insulin dose is reduced if the blood glucose is falling by > 100 mg/dl/hour.

✓ Blood glucose is measured hourly prior to each injection.

♥ Once blood glucose is ≤ 250 mg/dl, insulin is administered every 4-6 hours at 0.1-0.4 U/kg IM attempting to maintain the blood glucose concentration between 200 and 300 mg/dl.

♥ Dextrose should administered (5% dextrose) when the blood glucose is < 250 mg/dl with the rate adjusted to maintain the blood glucose at 200-300 mg/dl. It is preferable to administer the 5% dextrose as a separate infusion from the electrolyte solution as the infusion rate of the dextrose will be altered depending on the hourly blood glucose.

✓ Insulin can be administered SQ when hydration status is normal.

✔ Intermediate or long-acting insulin treatment can be instituted when the animal is eating normally.

✔ Low-dose IM treatment is effective in most cases, but requires hourly injections and blood glucose concentrations, necessitating considerable technical time.

Continuous Low-dose Intravenous Insulin Treatment

✔ Insulin dose is 2.2 U/kg/24 hours or 0.09 U/kg/hour in dogs, and 1.1 U/kg/24h or 0.045 U/kg/hr in cats as a constant rate IV infusion.

✔ Add the daily dose of regular insulin to 250 ml NaCl and allow 50 ml to flow through the IV administration set because insulin adheres to plastic.

✔ Initial infusion rate is 10 ml/hour using an infusion pump.

✔ Monitor blood glucose concentration hourly; less frequent monitoring (q 90 minutes is acceptable in most cases).

♥ When the blood glucose ≤ 250 mg/dl, decrease the infusion rate by 25-50% according to Table 10-1 and initiate dextrose administration in IV fluids.

✔ Begin intermediate or long-acting insulin when the animal is eating normally.

✔ Continuous low-dose IV insulin protocol is less labor intensive than the IM protocol since injections do not have to be given hourly and there is more leeway in the time of blood glucose monitoring.

✔ This is the authors' preferred treatment and works very predictably in dogs; more variation in response to insulin seems to occur in cats.

Table 10-1
Adjustment in Insulin and Dextrose Administration Using the Continuous Low-dose Intravenous Insulin Infusion Protocol

Blood Glucose Concentration (mg/dl)	IV Fluid Solution	Rate of IV Insulin Solution (ml/hour)*
>250	0.9% saline	10
200-250	0.45% saline, 2.5% dextrose	7
150-200	0.45% saline, 2.5% dextrose	5
100-150	0.45% saline, 5% dextrose	5
<100	0.45% saline, 5% dextrose	stop insulin infusion

*IV insulin solution contains 2.2 U/kg (dogs) or 1.1 U/Kg (cats) of regular insulin in 250 ml of 0.9% saline.
Adapted from: Macintire DK. Treatment of diabetic ketoacidosis in dogs by continuous low-dose intravenous infusion of insulin. J Am Vet Med Assoc 1993;202:1266-1272.

High-dose Intramuscular or Subcutaneous Insulin Treatment

✔ Insulin dose is 0.25-0.5 U/kg q 4 hours for IM, and 0.5 U/kg q 6 hours for SQ route.

✔ Subsequent dosage should be adjusted to maintain a blood glucose concentration of 200-300 mg/dl.

♥ 5% dextrose should be administered at a maintenance rate when the blood glucose < 250 mg/dl to maintain the blood glucose at 200-300 mg/dl.

✔ This protocol is simple and effective in most cases but carries a higher risk of hypoglycemia and hypokalemia because of the higher initial doses of insulin.

Bicarbonate Therapy

✔ The acidosis associated with diabetic ketoacidosis usually resolves after insulin administration and without supplemental sodium bicarbonate treatment.

♥ Bicarbonate treatment is rarely necessary.

✔ Side effects include worsening of hypokalemia, paradoxical CSF acidosis, and reduced ketone body metabolism.

♥ Treatment should be reserved for dogs and cats with an arterial or venous blood pH < 7.0 or with a plasma bicarbonate or total CO_2 concentration < 10 mEq/L.

✔ Sodium bicarbonate dose (mEq/L) = body weight (kg) x (24 − patient bicarbonate) x 0.4 x 0.25 (only 25% of the base deficit should be replaced by sodium bicarbonate initially).

✔ Further bicarbonate administration should be given only if severe acidosis continues to be present.

Phosphate Supplementation

♥ Severe hypophosphatemia results in hemolysis, muscle weakness, respiratory depression, cardiac dysfunction, and decreased tissue delivery of oxygen.

✔ Phosphate should be supplemented when the serum phosphorus concentration < 1.5 mg/dl.

✔ Potassium phosphate (initially 0.01 − 0 .03 mmol/kg/hr of phosphate administered in IV fluids) is used and will replace part of the potassium deficit as well. Serum phosphorus should be monitored at least twice per day during phosphate supplementation with dosage adjustments made to maintain normal phosphorus. Higher dosage rates may be necessary in some cases.

✔ Potassium phosphate is available as a solution containing 3 mmol/ml of phosphorus and 4.4 mEq/ml potassium.

✔ Side effects include hypocalcemia and soft tissue mineralization.

Potassium Supplementation

♥ Potassium deficit is almost always present even when serum potassium is normal.

✔ Treatment with IV fluids, insulin, and correction of acidosis will cause serum potassium to decrease.

✔ If serum potassium concentration is known, supplement according to Table 10-2.

✔ If serum potassium measurement is not immediately available, administer 40 mEq/L in IV fluids once adequate urine production has been documented.

💣 Monitor urine output to ensure that it is adequate and that acute renal failure has not occurred.

♥ Monitor serum potassium 3-4 hours after initiating fluid therapy when possible as hypokalemia often occurs soon after initiating fluids and insulin treatment. Subsequent monitoring of serum potassium should be considered every 8-12 hours with dosage adjustments as necessary to maintain normal serum potassium concentration.

Table 10-2
Potassium Supplementation in IV Fluids

Serum Potassium Concentration (mEq/L)	Potassium Supplement (mEq) in 1 Liter IV Fluids
3.5-5.0	20
3.0-3.5	30
2.5-3.0	40
2.0-2.5	60
<2.0	80

Do not exceed 0.5 mEq/kg/hour rate of potassium administration.

Supportive Care

♥ Identification and proper treatment of any underlying illness is crucial to the successful treatment of the dog or cat with diabetic ketoacidosis.

✔ Pancreatitis, infection, renal failure, and neoplasia are the most common concurrent diseases.

Long-term Treatment

✓ Once the animal is stable and eating, an intermediate or long-acting insulin can be administered as per standard care for uncomplicated diabetes mellitus.

✓ Insulin treatment may have to be altered as the underlying disease causing insulin resistance resolves.

Prognosis

✓ About 75% of dogs and cats survive initial treatment of diabetic ketoacidosis.

✓ The prognosis is usually dependent on the severity of underlying illness.

♥ Ketoacidosis reoccurs in many animals that survive the initial episode.

Non-ketotic Hyperosmolar Diabetes Mellitus

✓ A rare form of diabetes mellitus also called hyperglycemic hyperosmolar state.

♥ Severe hyperglycemia and dehydration without ketosis are hallmarks.

✓ Classical signs of diabetes mellitus are present in addition to lethargy, depression, anorexia, and weakness.

✓ Mental obtundation, stupor, or coma may be present.

✓ Laboratory abnormalities include blood glucose > 600 mg/dl, azotemia, variable serum electrolyte concentrations, and hyperosmolality.

✓ Serum osmolality can be calculated using the following formula:

$$\text{Osmolality} = 2(\text{Na}^+ + \text{K}^+) + \text{glucose}/18 + \text{BUN}/2.8$$

Normal osmolality (calculated) = 305-315 mOsm/kg

✓ Osmolality > 350 mOsm/kg can result in clinical signs and should prompt cautious treatment of hyperosmolality.

✓ Urine ketones are negative or present in a low concentration.

♥ Treatment is similar to that of diabetic ketoacidosis, with goals of a gradual decrease in blood glucose concentration (50-75 mg/dl/hour) being accomplished using either low-dose insulin protocol described for use in diabetic ketoacidosis.

💣 Cerebral edema is very possible if blood glucose is decreased too rapidly.

♥ Initially, 0.9% saline is administered for the first 4-6 hr. of treatment, followed by 0.45% saline.

♥ Urine output should be monitored closely, and 0.9% saline should be substituted for 0.45% saline if urine output is subnormal or if circulatory insufficiency is present as indicated by tachycardia, poor pulse quality, poor tissue perfusion, and hypotension.

✓ Electrolyte deficiencies are similar to those in diabetic ketoacidosis.

💣 Impaired renal function is often present, so potassium supplementation should be based on serial serum electrolyte measurements.

✓ Careful patient monitoring is crucial to detect oliguria, renal failure, circulatory collapse, cerebral edema, and electrolyte abnormalities common in this disease.

♥ Prognosis is poor with high mortality rates.

💣 Attempts should be made to not decrease serum sodium concentration more rapidly than 12 mEq/L/day.

Section 11
Hypoglycemia

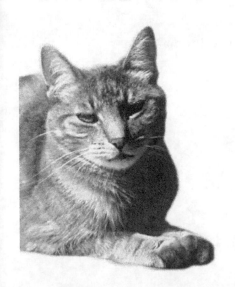

♥ Problems

Seizures

Coma

Stupor

Ataxia

Weakness

Muscle tremors

Exercise intolerance

Abnormal behavior

Increased appetite

Overview

✔ Hypoglycemia is a common finding on serum chemistries and it must initially be determined if the hypoglycemia is of significance or if it is either a variant of normal or a result of poor sample handling. Hypoglycemia in young animals is likely to be due to juvenile hypoglycemia, fasting, congenital liver disease, portosystemic shunts, or sepsis. Older animals are likely to have hypoglycemia due to neoplasia (insulinoma or non-islet cell tumor), acquired hepatic disease, hypoadrenocorticism, or sepsis. Treatment is directed at resolving the hypoglycemia if severe, then addressing the primary disease process.

Causes of Hypoglycemia

Insulin overdose

Insulin-secreting islet cell tumor (insulinoma)

Non-islet cell tumor

Sepsis

Hunting dog hypoglycemia

Hepatic failure

Hypoadrenocorticism

Neonatal hypoglycemia

Juvenile hypoglycemia

Preparturient hypoglycemia

Starvation

Error in sample handling or analysis

Clinical Signs

✓ Clinical signs depend on degree of hypoglycemia, duration (acute vs. chronic), cause, and age of the animal.

♥ Weakness, seizures, ataxia, collapse, and muscle tremors are the most common clinical signs.

♥ Bizarre behavior including apparent disorientation, "hysteria," nervousness, and irritability can occur.

✓ Dogs with insulinomas often gain weight due to the anabolic effects of insulin and increased food intake.

✓ Other signs include polyuria, polydipsia, syncope, exercise intolerance, and head tilt.

♥ Puppies with hypoglycemia may have stupor as the primary sign.

✓ Signs related to the primary disease process (sepsis, hepatic disease, etc.) may predominate.

♥ Physical examination may reveal the neurologic consequences of hypoglycemia, stimulation of the sympathetic nervous system (tachycardia), or abnormalities related to the primary disease process. Non-islet cell tumors are usually large and palpable abdominal tumors. Dogs with insulinoma usually have no physical examination abnormalities other than those attributable to hypoglycemia. Dogs with sepsis, hepatic failure, and hypoadrenocorticism usually have a variety of abnormalities on exam.

Routine Laboratory Tests

✓ Finding hypoglycemia will provide an explanation of clinical signs and distinguish it from other differential diagnoses including hypocalcemia, primary CNS disease, and hepatic encephalopathy.

✍ Hypoglycemia should be confirmed by repeat analysis.

♥ Routine complete blood count, serum chemistries (including electrolytes), and urinalysis will identify evidence of many disorders causing hypoglycemia including hepatic failure, hypoadrenocorticism, and sepsis.

✓ Hepatic failure is usually accompanied by decreased albumin, BUN, and possibly cholesterol, as well as elevated liver enzymes. Dogs with portosystemic shunts may have few biochemical abnormalities.

✓ Hypoadrenocorticism typically results in hyperkalemia, hyponatremia, hypochloremia, and metabolic acidosis.

♥ Atypical hypoadrenocorticism and withdrawal of glucocorticoids after prolonged use will result in an isolated glucocorticoid deficiency and plasma electrolytes will be normal. Hypoglycemia may be the primary clinical finding in these patients.

✓ Sepsis is usually readily identified by history, physical examination, typical hemogram abnormalities, and frequently, urinary tract infection.

✋ Use of hand-held glucometers may result in a falsely decreased blood glucose reading by the nature of the device. Sample size must be adequate when using these devices, otherwise the blood glucose will be falsely low.

Diagnostic Imaging

✓ Hepatic, splenic, and gastrointestinal masses (non-islet cell neoplasia) are readily identified on abdominal radiographs or ultrasound.

✓ Hepatic diseases including cirrhosis, hepatitis, and portosystemic shunt may be identified on abdominal ultrasound.

✓ Insulinoma can sometimes be identified on ultrasound examination as a mass in the pancreas (Figure 11-1), abdominal lymph node enlargement, or multiple hepatic masses representing metastasis.

✓ Identification of a locus of infection (i.e. pneumonia on radiographs, pyelonephritis on ultrasound) may be found in cases of sepsis.

✓ Megaesophagus is occasionally present on thoracic radiographs in dogs with hypoadrenocorticism.

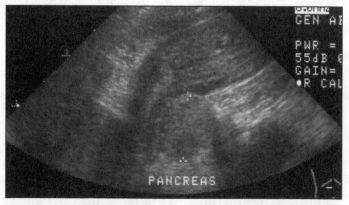

Figure 11-1 Insulinoma identified as a hypoechoic mass in the pancreas located between the markers. (Courtesy Dr. Martha Moon-Larsen)

Specific Tests for Diagnosis

♥ History, physical examination, confirmation of hypoglycemia, and response to treatment is adequate for diagnosis of neonatal hypoglycemia and juvenile hypoglycemia.

♥ Concurrent disease causing anorexia may precipitate hypoglycemia in young animals.

✓ Liver function testing such as pre- and post-prandial bile acids should be abnormal if hepatic failure is causing the hypoglycemia. Liver function should be evaluated in all dogs with any evidence of hepatic disease prior to measurement of insulin.

✓ An ACTH response test should find low plasma cortisol concentration in response to ACTH if hypoadrenocorticism is present.

✓ Identification of an elevated or inappropriately normal fasting plasma insulin concentration with concurrent hypoglycemia is diagnostic of insulinoma. The blood sample must be collected after fasting and while the blood glucose is less than 60 mg/dl, preferably even lower. This test should be reserved for cases where other causes of hypoglycemia have been ruled out.

Treatment Recommendations

Emergency Treatment of Hypoglycemic Crisis

℞ Administration of 1 ml/kg 50% dextrose (diluted to a 25% or less solution if possible) as an intravenous bolus. This dose can be repeated 2-3 times until effective or if clinical signs recur.

♥ Following resolution of signs of hypoglycemia in response to the dextrose bolus, IV fluids with 2.5 to 5% dextrose are administered.

♥ Blood glucose should initially be monitored hourly and maintained between 60-150 mg/dl.

♥ Some animals, particularly those suffering an insulin overdose or with insulinoma, may require a higher concentration of dextrose (10-20%) to maintain euglycemia.

✓ Dextrose solutions > 10% may cause phlebitis and should not be given for prolonged periods in a peripheral vein.

✓ If brain injury is present due to prolonged, severe hypoglycemia, caution should be taken to avoid hyperglycemia as it may worsen the CNS damage.

♥ If hypoglycemia persists despite appropriate IV dextrose administration, glucagon can be administered as a constant rate infusion. The initial dose rate is 5 ng/kg/min, which can be increased in 5 ng/kg/min increments up to 20 ng/kg/min or higher as necessary to maintain the blood glucose >60 mg/dl.

♥ Persistence of neurologic signs after resolution of the hypoglycemia likely indicates neuroglucopenic damage to the brain. It can result in temporary or permanent neurologic deficits including coma, blindness, ataxia, and behavioral changes. A glucocorticoid (dexamethasone sodium phosphate 1-2 mg/kg IV), mannitol (0.5-1.0 g/kg IV over 20 minutes), and furosemide (1-2 mg/kg IV) can be administered for treatment of cerebral edema, but are unlikely to have much effect.

Management of Non-emergent Hypoglycemia

♥ Frequent feeding of puppies and juvenile small dogs will prevent hypoglycemia.

✓ Resolution of concurrent disease of puppies should prevent future episodes.

♥ If hypoglycemia is induced by insulin administration at the prescribed dose, the dosage should be decreased by 25-50%. Insulin should not be administered until it is clear that the effect of the last dose has waned and hyperglycemia has resulted. Reasons for the hypoglycemia should be investigated, including diet change, increase in exercise, new bottle of insulin, and change in type of insulin.

✓ Surgical excision of the tumor, when possible, is the treatment of choice for non-islet cell neoplasms. Leiomyosarcomas of the gastrointestinal tract are particularly amenable to surgery.

Prognosis

✓ Dependent on cause of hypoglycemia. When the underlying cause can be effectively treated, hypoglycemia should resolve.

Insulinoma

Overview

✓ Insulinoma is uncommon in the dog and rare in the cat.

♥ Insulinomas are usually malignant and have gross evidence of metastasis to regional lymph node or liver in about 50% of dogs at the time of surgery.

Clinical Signs

✓ Signs of hypoglycemia as described previously.

✓ Weight gain, increased appetite, and obesity may occur due to the anabolic effects of insulin excess.

✓ Generalized weakness and hyporeflexia due to peripheral neuropathy are occasionally present.

Routine Laboratory Tests

♥ Hypoglycemia is usually very severe, but is dependent on duration of fasting prior to sampling.

✓ Elevations of alkaline phosphatase and ALT activity are common.

Diagnostic Imaging

✓ A pancreatic mass can be identified on abdominal ultrasound in 1/3-1/2 of cases (see Figure 11-1).

Specific Tests for Diagnosis

☞ Measurement of fasting blood glucose and serum insulin concentrations concurrently.

☞ A normal or elevated serum insulin concentration with concurrent hypoglycemia (preferably a blood glucose <50 mg/dl) is diagnostic for insulinoma.

✋ Failure to identify another cause for severe, persistent hypo-glycemia in an older dog despite a thorough search (including ACTH response test, liver function test) makes insulinoma highly likely.

Treatment

✋ Surgery with partial pancreatectomy removing the insulinoma and excision of visible metastases is the treatment of choice. It may prolong the period of hypoglycemia even if the tumor is not completely excised.

♥ Abnormalities suspected to be hepatic metastasis based on ultrasound examination or visualization at surgery may be nodular regeneration or hepatomas, so one must be very cautious about concluding that metastatic disease is present without histopathologic confirmation.

♥ Surgery should be performed by an experienced surgeon and 24 hour postoperative care should be available. Intraoperative and postoperative blood glucose monitoring is critical.

♥ Complications in the perioperative period include pancreatitis, hypoglycemia, hyperglycemia, and sepsis.

♥ Medical management is indicated if owners decline surgery or if signs persist or recur despite surgery.

♥ Frequent feedings (4-6 times daily) of a food with minimal simple sugar content and restriction of exercise should be attempted as a method to reduce severity of hypoglycemia prior to other medical management.

♥ Glucocorticoids are administered when dietary management fails. Prednisone is initially given at 0.25 mg/kg BID, with the dosage increased incrementally up to 2 mg/kg BID as necessary to control signs of hypoglycemia.

♥ Diazoxide inhibits insulin release and can be effective in managing dogs with insulinomas that become refractory to prednisone and dietary management. Treatment is begun at 5 mg/kg PO BID and increased in 5 mg/kg increments up to 30 mg/kg BID as necessary to control hypoglycemia. Diazoxide is very costly and availability is limited.

✓ Octreotide is a somatostatin analog that inhibits insulin secretion. It has been used with limited success in a few cases of insulinoma, but it is expensive and must be given by subcutaneous injection. Dosages range from 10-50 µg per dose to 2-4 µg/kg BID or TID.

✓ Cytotoxic chemotherapy using streptozocin has been used, although its efficacy appears somewhat low. Streptozocin is nephrotoxic and less commonly hepatotoxic. An intensive diuresis protocol similar to that used for administration of cisplatin has been used to reduce the nephrotoxicity to an acceptable risk.

Prognosis

♥ Overall median survival of dogs treated surgically for insulinoma is about 1 year.

✓ Dogs with distant metastasis have shorter survival than dogs without detectable metastasis.

✓ Median survival for dogs treated medically is 2-3 months.

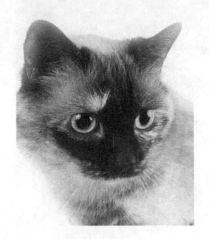

Section 12
Hypercalcemia

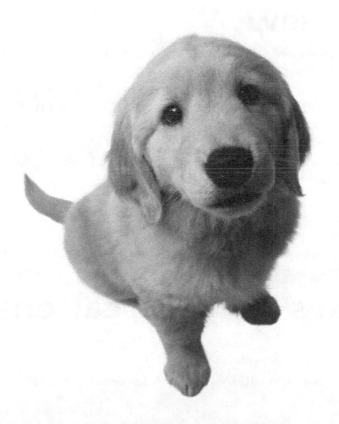

♥ Problems

Polydipsia/polyuria

Seizures

Anorexia

Vomiting

Diarrhea

Constipation

Twitching

Urolithiasis

Urinary tract infections

Mental dullness/lethargy

Muscle weakness

Soft tissue mineralization

Azotemia

Isosthenuria

Overview

♥ Calcium plays a vital role in homeostasis and is intimately involved with muscle and nerve function.

♥ The biologically active form of calcium is the ionized portion, although much is protein-bound (35-40%). Calcium (10% normally) also circulates complexed with anions such as citrate, bicarbonate, and phosphate.

✓ Elevation of ionized calcium has a negative feedback effect on parathyroid hormone (PTH) production. This is a very tightly regulated feedback loop.

✓ Ionized hypercalcemia is responsible for the majority of clinical signs.

✓ There are many causes of hypercalcemia in both dogs and cats. Treatment is directed at the underlying cause when possible.

Causes of Hypercalcemia

Laboratory error

Hypercalcemia of malignancy

Hypoadrenocorticism (30 to 40% of Addisonian patients are hypercalcemic)

Dehydration

Primary hyperparathyroidism

Renal failure

Granulomatous disease (Blastomycosis, Coccidiodomycosis, Schistosomiasis)

Osteomyelitis

Bone neoplasia

Cholecalciferol rodenticide intoxication

Hypervitaminosis D

Normal variation in juvenile animals

Idiopathic hypercalcemia in cats

Diagnostic Approach

♥ Over 40% of all cases of hypercalcemia in dogs and <30% in cats are caused by hypercalcemia of malignancy.

✓ Lymphosarcoma (especially mediastinal forms in dogs), apocrine gland adenocarcinoma of the anal sac, and multiple myeloma are the most common causes in the dog.

✓ Lymphosarcoma and squamous cell carcinoma are the most common causes of hypercalcemia of malignancy in cats.

✓ Renal failure is a common cause of hypercalcemia in dogs and cats; approximately 10% of patients with renal failure are hypercalcemic.

✓ Idiopathic hypercalcemia is a common cause of mild to moderate hypercalcemia in cats.

History and Physical Examination

✓ The lymph nodes should be carefully palpated for enlargement that could be associated with lymphosarcoma or granulomatous disease.

✓ A rectal examination to identify an anal sac mass or metastasis to the sublumbar lymph nodes is warranted.

✓ A thorough history should be taken to rule out vitamin D supplementation or access to cholecalciferol rodenticides or medications such as calcipotriene.

✔ Abdominal palpation may reveal small kidneys with renal failure or organomegaly secondary to neoplasia.

✔ Palpate the neck carefully for a parathyroid mass, particularly in cats.

Common Clinical Signs

General

☛ Clinical signs are often not apparent until total calcium is above 15 mg/dL.

☛ In those cases where hypercalcemia is attributable to neoplasia, renal failure or hypoadrenocorticism the clinical signs of the underlying disease may predominate over signs attributable to the elevated calcium.

♥ Lethargy.

♥ Weakness.

✔ Widespread soft tissue mineralization, especially if hypercalcemia and hyperphosphatemia are present.

Renal/Urinary

♥ Polyuria/polydipsiaare the most common clinical signs of hypercalcemia in dogs. Polyuria occurs because hypercalcemia impairs the response of the collecting tubules to antidiuretic hormone.

✔ Renal insufficiency/failure can be caused by persistent hypercalcemia, which leads to renal vasoconstriction and nephrocalcinosis.

☛ Because azotemia and isosthenuria can occur secondary to hypercalcemia without substantial irreversible renal damage, renal failure is difficult or impossible to diagnose in some hypercalcemic animals. Evaluation of renal function following resolution of the hypercalcemia is the only reliable method of determining the presence of renal failure in some cases.

✔ Calcium urolithiasis occurs in 30% of dogs with primary hyperparathyroidism.

✔ Bacterial urinary tract infections are common.

Cardiovascular

✔ Premature beats, especially of ventricular origin can occur.

✔ Shortened QT interval.

Gastrointestinal

♥ Anorexia is the most common clinical sign of hypercalcemia in cats.

✓ Vomiting and diarrhea can occur.

✓ Constipation is sometimes seen.

✓ Severe bloody gastroenteritis can occur in the initial phase of cholecalciferol toxicity.

✓ Pancreatitis is suspected to be associated with hypercalcemia in some patients, although it is rare and poorly documented.

Neurologic

✓ Seizures can occur and relate to hyperpolarization of the neuronal cell membranes.

♥ Twitching, shivering, or stiff gait can be neuromuscular manifestations of hypercalcemia.

Routine Laboratory Tests

Complete Blood Count

✓ Neoplastic cells, especially lymphocytes can be seen in some cases of lymphoma or leukemia.

✓ Cytopenias may be indicative of bone marrow disease.

Serum Chemistries

✓ Hyperkalemia and hyponatremia may indicate hypoadrenocorticism.

✓ Azotemia may indicate renal disease, especially if hyperphosphatemia is present. With hypercalcemia azotemia can be pre-renal or renal in origin.

✓ Hyperglobulinemia may indicate multiple myeloma. Serum electrophoresis should demonstrate a monoclonal gammopathy.

♥ Total calcium consists of a protein bound, complexed (usually to phosphates or other anions) and an ionized fraction. Total calcium values are influenced by the albumin concentration. The following formula will correct for various albumin levels: adjusted calcium (mg/dL) = measured calcium (mg/dL) − measured albumin (g/dL) + 3.5. This calculation is not valid in cats.

✓ The normal reference range for calcium is higher in young animals.

✔ Ionized calcium measures the biologically active form of calcium. Elevations in ionized calcium can be seen with hypercalcemia of malignancy, primary hyperparathyroidism or hypervitaminosis D. Measuring ionized calcium is indicated in any patient with repeatable elevations of total calcium.

✔ Phosphorus: In those cases where hypercalcemia results from excess PTH or PTH-RP, calcium will be high and phosphorus typically low or low-normal. In animals with renal failure associated hypercalcemia phosphorus is usually elevated. It may be difficult to differentiate renal failure with hypercalcemia from hypercalcemia induced renal failure.

✔ The normal reference range for phosphorus is higher in young animals.

Urinalysis

✔ Minimally concentrated urine is common with hypercalcemia.

✔ Does not necessarily indicate impaired renal function.

♥ Bacterial urinary tract infections are common; a culture may be warranted in most animals that are hypercalcemic.

Further Diagnostic Tests

♥ Because hypercalcemia of malignancy is a common cause of hypercalcemia, considerable effort should be directed toward search for neoplasia.

✔ Lymph node aspirates or biopsies are indicated to rule out lymphoma.

✔ Bone marrow aspiration/biopsy may be indicated to rule out neoplasia. If cytopenias or a gammopathy is present this becomes more likely to be a useful test.

✔ Transtracheal wash, bronchoalveolar lavage, or lung aspiration may be needed to diagnose pulmonary fungal infections.

✔ An ACTH stimulation test is needed to diagnose hypoadrenocorticism.

Diagnostic Imaging

Radiographs

✓ Thoracic radiographs should be obtained for evidence of metastatic disease or a mediastinal mass. Granulomatous disease (i.e. fungal infections) can also be seen on thoracic radiographs.

✓ Abdominal radiographs are useful in detecting tumors. The area of the sublumbar lymph nodes should be closely investigated (metastasis from an anal sac adenocarcinoma).

✓ Abdominal radiographs will help to identify urolithiasis.

✓ Radiographs of the skeleton may identify lytic lesions consistent with neoplasia (multiple myeloma).

✓ Osteopenia may be evident, especially apparent with skull radiographs (Figure 12-1).

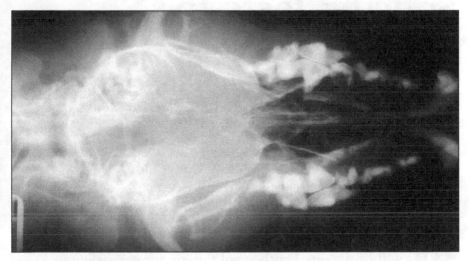

Figure 12-1 Skull radiographs demonstrating severe osteopenia secondary to prolonged primary hyperparathyroidism in a Keeshond.

Ultrasonography

✓ Ultrasonograph of the neck may be able to reveal a mass with primary hyperparathyroidism (Figure 12-2).

✓ Ultrasonography of the abdomen can help to find tumors or lymph node enlargement.

✓ Thoracic ultrasound can help to define mediastinal masses.

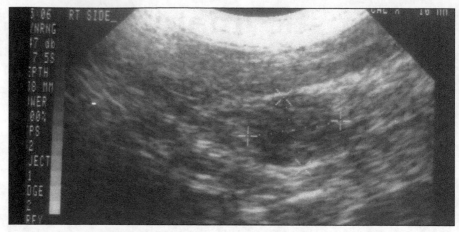

Figure 12-2 Ultrasound of the thyroparathyroid area with a hypoechoic parathyroid mass delineated by markers.

Specific Tests for Diagnosis

PTH (Intact Parathyroid Hormone)

PTH analysis is indicated in any patient with ionized hypercalcemia if initial diagnostics fail to find a cause such as a neoplasm.

✓ Parathyroid hormone increases calcium concentration by reducing urinary excretion, increasing bone resorption and increasing formation of active vitamin D.

♥ Elevated or high normal PTH in the face of ionized hypercalcemia without renal failure is strongly suggestive of primary hyperparathyroidism.

♥ PTH will be elevated with renal failure; ionized calcium, however, is usually low or in the normal range.

✓ Low PTH in the face of ionized hypercalcemia suggests either hypercalcemia of malignancy or granulomatous disease related hypercalcemia.

PTH-RP (PTH Related Protein)

✓ Similar effects as PTH but is formed by tumor cells. Elevated PTH-RP with low PTH and ionized hypercalcemia is consistent with hypercalcemia of malignancy.

✋ PTHrP is not elevated in all cases of hypercalcemia of malignancy.

Vitamin D

✓ Can be elevated in granulomatous disease.

✓ Elevated with vitamin D toxicosis.

✓ Measurement of 25-hydroxycholecalciferol or calcitriol is infrequently indicated when evaluating hypercalcemia.

Treatment Recommendations

☞ Primary efforts in managing hypercalcemia should be directed toward treatment of the underlying cause This may require surgery for primary hyperparathyroidism or some tumors, chemotherapy for neoplasia, or antifungal therapy if related to an infection such as blastomycosis.

💣 Indications for aggressive treatment of hypercalcemia include dehydration, azotemia, serum calcium >16 mg/dl, a calcium x phosphorus product > 70, a rapidly increasing serum calcium concentration, or significant clinical signs of hypercalcemia. Failure to lower the calcium in these situations can lead to serious and irreversible complications including renal failure.

♥ Fluid therapy, preferably using 0.9% NaCl, initially aims to correct dehydration and to expand the intravascular volume. Diuresis helps to increase renal excretion of calcium and maintain renal perfusion. Fluids should be part of the therapeutic plan in all hypercalcemic animals that require aggressive treatment unless otherwise contraindicated.

✓ Furosemide (2-4 mg/kg IV or IM) can be used in more severe cases since it inhibits calcium resorption in the kidney. Only use with concurrent fluid therapy.

💣 Prednisone can be used to reduce calcium resorption. It will, however, potentially alter cytology of tumors, especially lymphoma making a definitive diagnosis difficult. It is a relatively common, sometimes effective therapy for idiopathic hypercalcemia of cats.

✓ Sodium bicarbonate can be used if acidosis is present. Generally 1 to 2 mEq/kg is administered initially.

✓ Calcitonin (4-6 units/kg SQ BID/TID) is usually effective and has a rapid onset of action. It is expensive, has GI side effects, and is effective for only a few days.

✔ Biphosphonates are inhibitors of bone resorption. Pamidronate disodium (1 mg/kg given as a 2 hour IV infusion) is effective in dogs with hypercalcemia of malignancy and vitamin D toxicity. A single dose has an onset of action of 24 to 72 hours and a duration of effect of 1 to 4 weeks. It should be used with caution in dogs with impaired renal function.

✔ Plicamycin (mithramycin) is rarely used because side effects can be severe (bone marrow suppression, renal toxicity, liver toxicity).

Prognosis

✔ Dependent on the primary disease causing the hypercalcemia.

✔ Generally very good if primary disease can be treated effectively.

✔ Renal failure and damage caused by soft tissue mineralization may be permanent.

Primary Hyperparathyroidism

Overview

✔ Usually caused by functional adenomas of one of the parathyroid glands, though occasionally carcinomas can occur.

✔ Hyperplasia of multiple parathyroid glands is an occasional cause of primary hyperparathyroidism.

✔ Generally seen in older animals

✔ Possible breed predilection in Keeshonds

Clinical Signs

✔ Clinical signs relate to hypercalcemia as outlined above though these animals are rarely ill.

✔ An enlarged parathyroid gland is frequently palpable in cats but not in dogs.

✔ Urolithiasis and urinary tract infections are very common.

Routine Laboratory Tests

♥ Hypercalcemia is always present, usually marked (>13 mg/dL), and serum phosphorus is usually below or at the lower end of the reference range.

✓ Urinalysis often shows isosthenuria.

✓ UTI are common

Specific Tests for Diagnosis

♥ An elevated to high normal PTH, negative PTH-RP and ionized hypercalcemia are consistent with primary hyperparathyroidism.

Treatment

✓ Fluid therapy is indicated if the patient is dehydrated, azotemia is present, or serum calcium is markedly elevated.

✓ Surgery to remove the abnormal parathyroid tissue is indicated (Figure 12-3).

✓ During surgery all enlarged parathyroids are removed.

♥ Unaffected parathyroid glands in a patient with a single parathyroid gland adenoma will be small due to atrophy.

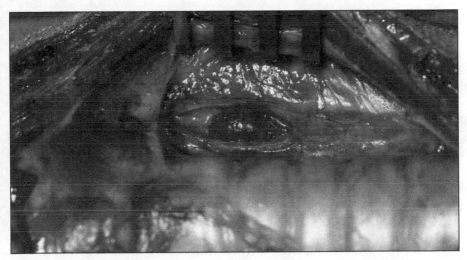

Figure 12-3 Unilateral parathyroid gland adenoma in a Great Dane with primary hyperparathyroidism.

✓ If the parathyroid glands are all of similar size in a dog where primary hyperparathyroidism has been confirmed, the diagnosis is likely parathyroid gland hyperplasia. In this case, 3 of 4 parathyroid glands are removed.

✓ After surgery the normal, suppressed parathyroid glands will eventually resume their function.

💣 Hypocalcemia commonly occurs after parathyroidectomy. Serum calcium should be measured daily for 3-5 days after surgery.

Prompt intervention is needed to avoid severe problems.

💣 Postoperative hypocalcemia is most common in patients with a presurgical calcium concentration > 14 mg/dL.

♥ Vitamin D treatment is recommended immediately postoperatively in dogs with a serum calcium > 14 mg/dl.

✓ Dihydrotachysterol is administered at an initial loading dose of 0.015 mg/kg PO BID for 2 days followed by 0.01 mg/kg BID for 2 days, followed by a maintenance dose of 0.01 mg/kg daily.

✋ Management of hypocalcemia is discussed more thoroughly in Section 13. Goal is to maintain calcium in the lower range of normal. This will stimulate the suppressed parathyroid glands to become functional again so treatment can be gradually tapered and discontinued after 6-8 weeks.

Section 13
Hypocalcemia

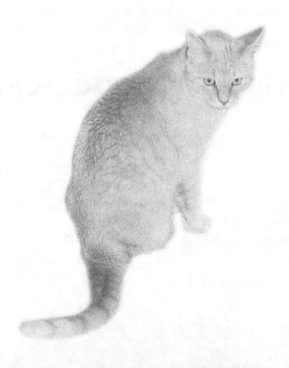

♥ Problems

Tetany

Seizures

Stiff gait

Muscle fasciculations

Weakness

Cataracts

Facial rubbing

Protrusion of nictitating membranes

Ptyalism

Panting

Hyperthermia

Anorexia

Overview

Hypocalcemia is a common biochemical abnormality in dogs and cats, caused by numerous conditions. Hypocalcemia sufficient to result in clinical signs occurs infrequently, and is usually due to puerperal tetany, iatrogenic hypoparathyroidism, or primary hypoparathyroidism. Treatment, when necessary, typically involves calcium administration with or without vitamin D supplementation.

Causes of Hypocalcemia

Puerperal tetany

Hypoparathyroidism (spontaneous or iatrogenic)

Renal failure

Pancreatitis

Ethylene glycol intoxication

Phosphate containing enema administration

Hypoalbuminemia

Urethral obstruction

Transfusion of blood with excessive citrate

Alkalosis

Clinical Signs

♥ Tetany can be localized, resulting in muscle spasms, and is sometimes induced by exercise. Stiff gait, weakness, muscle fasciculations, and generalized tremors can occur.

♥ Facial rubbing or pawing is common, probably secondary to cramping of facial muscles.

♥ Generalized seizures may occur spontaneously or after handling.

✓ Behavioral changes including restlessness and aggression are common in dogs.

✓ Hyperthermia secondary to increased muscle contractions.

✓ Cataracts may occur after prolonged hypocalcemia and are located in the anterior and posterior cortical subcapsular area of the lens.

✓ Cats may have ptyalism and protruding nictitating membranes in addition to other signs.

✓ Panting or hyperventilation is common.

✓ Anorexia, lethargy, vomiting, and diarrhea are occasionally found.

✓ Other clinical signs related to the primary disease process may be present.

✓ Puerperal tetany usually occurs postpartum, but can occur near the end of pregnancy.

Routine Laboratory Tests

✓ Total calcium should be corrected for hypoalbuminemia in dogs if appropriate (corrected calcium = 3.5 − patient albumin in g/dl + patient calcium in mg/dl).

✓ Confirming hypocalcemia using ionized calcium is usually unnecessary.

✓ Hyperphosphatemia may be present in primary hypoparathyroidism, renal failure, and phosphate enema toxicity.

✓ Renal azotemia is present in renal failure or late in ethylene glycol toxicosis.

✓ Elevated amylase and lipase as well as other clinicopathologic changes may occur with acute pancreatitis.

Diagnostic Imaging

✓ Indicated for specific diseases causing hypocalcemia such as pancreatitis, renal failure, etc.

Specific Tests for Diagnosis

✓ Ionized calcium can be measured in selected cases, but usually decreased total calcium and clinical signs are sufficient for confirming clinically significant hypocalcemia.

♥ History and physical examination often provide the most information regarding the etiology of hypocalcemia.

✓ Serum parathyroid hormone (PTH) is used when primary hypoparathyroidism is suspected. Serum PTH concentration should be low or low normal in the presence of hypocalcemia and often hyperphosphatemia.

Treatment Recommendations

✋ Calcium solutions have different calcium contents:

Calcium gluconate: 10% solution has 9.3 mg calcium/ml

Calcium chloride: 10% solution has 27.2 mg calcium/ml

♥ Calcium gluconate is preferred because it is less irritating if extravasation occurs.

Emergency Treatment of Tetany or Seizures

🩺 IV administration of calcium gluconate (10% solution; 1-1.5 ml/kg over 10-20 minutes) with close monitoring (including ECG) for bradycardia, vomiting, shortened QT interval, and elevated ST segment. If side effects occur, infusion should be stopped and reinstituted at a lower dose or administration rate when they resolve.

✓ The response to treatment should be prompt, but some clinical signs may not completely resolve for up to an hour after calcium administration.

♥ The initial IV bolus of calcium is followed with a constant rate infusion of calcium gluconate (6-10 ml/kg calcium gluconate/24 hours), additional boluses of calcium gluconate (1.5-2 ml/kg 10% solution q 6-8 hr) or by subcutaneous administration of calcium gluconate.

💣 Calcium gluconate must be diluted with sterile saline (1:1 or preferably more dilute) prior to subcutaneous injection; there have been a limited number of reports of severe tissue mineralization caused by SQ administration of calcium gluconate.

💣 Calcium chloride should never be administered subcutaneously as it is very irritating.

Management of Non-emergent Hypocalcemia

🔑 A combination of oral calcium and vitamin D preparations are used when long-term hypocalcemia is anticipated, as in primary hypoparathyroidism.

✓ Oral calcium is administered initially at 25-50 mg elemental calcium per day.

✓ Calcium carbonate is 40% calcium, calcium lactate is 13% calcium, and calcium gluconate is 10% calcium.

✓ Oral calcium supplementation can often be discontinued after vitamin D treatment has taken effect.

✓ Vitamin D preparations are used to increase intestinal absorption of calcium.

♥ Dihydrotachysterol and calcitriol are the preferred preparations as they have a relatively rapid onset of action and relatively short duration of action.

🖐 The duration of effect is important because toxicity due to overdose can cause hypercalcemia and hyperphosphatemia.

♥ Dihydrotachysterol has a maximal effect in 1-7 days and a duration of effect of 1-3 weeks. Dosage is 0.02-0.03 mg/kg/day for 2-3 days, then 0.01-0.02 q 24-48 hours.

♥ Calcitriol has a maximal effect in 1-4 days and a duration of effect of 2-7 days. Dosage is 20-30 ng/kg/day for 3-4 days, then 5-15 ng/kg/day, divided twice daily.

🔑 Dosages of vitamin D compounds are adjusted to maintain the serum calcium at or just below the lower limit of the normal range. Calcium should be monitored daily during the initial treatment until the calcium nears the low normal range. Weekly measurements should then be taken until a stable serum calcium concentration is reached, then every 3 months.

💣※ Hypercalcemia is a serious side effect of calcium and vitamin D supplementation. Renal failure and other consequences of hypercalcemia can occur if prolonged or severe hypercalcemia develops because of oversupplemenation of vitamin D compounds.

♥ Animals with puerperal tetany should be administered supplemental oral calcium for the duration of lactation. Weaning should be considered if signs of hypocalcemia are recurrent.

✔ The vitamin D dosage can be decreased gradually over a 6-8 week period in cases where parathyroid or thyroid surgery has caused hypocalcemia.

Prognosis

✔ Dependent on the primary disease causing the hypocalcemia.

✔ Puerperal tetany has an excellent prognosis, but recurrence in subsequent pregnancies is possible.

✔ With proper management, particularly avoiding hypercalcemia, the prognosis of primary hypoparathyroidism is good.

Primary Hypoparathyroidism

Overview

✔ Uncommon disease caused by destruction of parathyroid glands, usually secondary to lymphocytic parathyroiditis.

✔ Iatrogenic hypoparathyroidism occurs after bilateral parathyroidectomy, most often associated with thyroidectomy.

Clinical Signs

✔ Occurs at any age, but young adult dogs are frequently affected.

✔ Clinical signs are related to hypocalcemia as described above.

✔ Signs of hypocalcemia are intermittent in most cases, and may be induced by exercise or stress.

Routine Laboratory Tests

♥ Hypocalcemia is always present and the serum calcium concentration may be extremely low.

✓ Hyperphosphatemia is present in almost all cases.

Specific Tests for Diagnosis

♥ Serum PTH concentration below normal or in the low-normal range despite severe hypocalcemia is diagnostic of primary hypoparathyroidism.

Treatment

✓ Long-term treatment with some form of vitamin D with or without calcium supplementation as described above.

✋ It is crucial to avoid hypercalcemia.

Appendix 1

Questionnaire for Patients with Diabetes

Patient name: _____

Date _____

Type of insulin administered: _____

Time and dose of last insulin: Time _____Dose _____

Diet and amount fed: Diet _____Amount _____

Time of last meal and amount eaten: _____

Water intake:	Decreased	Normal	Increased
Urine production:	Decreased	Normal	Increased
Appetite:	Decreased	Normal	Increased
Stamina and strength:	Decreased	Normal	Increased

Have you had any problem with injections? _____

Have you noticed any signs of hypoglycemia including
weakness, loss of balance, behavior changes, seizures?   Yes   No

Other complications/concerns: _____

Appendix 2
Endocrine Drugs
Pituitary

DDAVP
    DDAVP intranasal preparation: 100 μg/ml, Rhone-Poulenc Rorer
    Pharmaceuticals; Stimate (Centeon) 1.5 mg/ml
    DDAVP Tablets: 0.1 and 0.2 mg, Rhone-Poulenc Rorer
    Pharmaceuticals
    DDAVP Injection: 15 μg/ml and 4 μg/ml, Rhone-Poulenc Rorer
    Pharmaceuticals

Vasopressin (ADH)
    Vasopressin (8-arginine vasopressin): 20 units/ml, various manufacturers
    Pitressin: 20 units/ml, 1 ml vial, Monarch

Growth hormone
    Various preparations and manufacturers

Thyroid

Levothyroxine
    Various manufacturers

Liothyronine
    Cytomel: 5, 25, 50 μg tablets, Monarch
    Triostat: injectable 10 μg/ml in 1 ml vial, Monarch

Methimazole
    Tapazole: 5 and 10 mg tablets, King

Propylthiouracil
    50 mg tablets, various manufacturers

Carbimazole
    Neomercazole, Roche

Iopanoic acid
    Telepaque: 500 mg tablets

Potassium iodide
    Thyroblock: 130 mg tablets, Wallace

TRH
    Relefact TRH: 500 μg vial, Ferring; Thyrel TRH: 500 μg vial, Ferring;
    Thypione: 500 μg vial, Abbott

TSH
    Thyrotropin-alpha (human recombinant TSH): Thyrogen: 1.1 mg
    ($\geq$ 4 IU) vial, Genzyme

Pancreas

Insulins
  Various preparations and manufacturers; see Section 9

Vetsulin
  Porcine insulin zinc suspension (Lente): 40 U/ml, Intervet

PZI Vet
  Protamine zinc insulin, IDEXX

Potassium phosphate
  Various manufacturers

Potassium chloride
  Various manufacturers

Octreotide
  Sandostatin: 0.05-5 mg/ml, Novartis
  Sandostatin LAR Depot: 10-30 mg/5 ml, Novartis

Metformin
  Glucophage: 500, 800, 1000 mg tablets, Bristol-Myers Squibb

Diazoxide
  Proglycem: 50 mg capsule, 50 mg/ml oral suspension, Baker-Norton

Streptozocin
  Zonosar: 100 mg/ml, 1 g vial, Upjohn Co.

Glucagon
  Glucagon Emergency Kit: 1 mg in syringe, Eli Lily

Glipizide
  Glucotrol: 5 mg tablets, Pfizer; various manufacturers

Glyburide
  DiaBeta: 1.25 mg tablets, Hoechst Marion Roussel; various
  manufacturers

Acarbose
  Precose: 50, 100 mg tablets, Bayer

Adrenal

Mitotane
  Lysodren: 500 mg tablets, Bristol-Myers Oncology/Immunology

Deprenyl
  Anipryl: 2, 10, 30 mg tablets, Pfizer Animal Health

Ketoconazole
  Nizoral: 200 mg capsule, Janssen
  Various manufacturers

Trilostane
   Vetoryl: 30 mg capsule, Arnolds Veterinary Products Ltd.

Glucocorticoids
   Various preparations and manufacturers
   Dexamethasone
   Dexamethasone sodium phosphate
   Prednisone
   Prednisolone
   Hydrocortisone sodium phosphate
   Hydrocortone phosphate: 50 mg/ml, MSD

Fludrocortisone
   Florinef Acetate: 0.1 mg tablets, Apothecon

Desoxycorticosterone pivilate
   Percorten: 25 mg/ml in 4 ml vial, Novartis Animal Health

ACTH
   Cosyntropin; Cortrosyn: 0.25 mg vial, Amphastar

Metyrapone
   Metopirone: 250 mg capsule, Novartis

Aminoglutethimide
   Cytadren: 250 mg tablets, Ciba Pharmaceutical Co

Calcium

Calcitonin
   Calcimar: 200 IU, Rhone-Poulenc Rorer; Osteocalcin, Arcola;
   Salmonine, Lennod

Pamidronate
   Aredia: 30, 90 mg injectable, Novartis

Aledronate
   Fosamax: 5-70 mg tablets, Merck

Etidronate
   Didronel: 200, 400 mg tablets, Procter & Gamble Pharmaceutical

Calcitriol
   Rocatraol: 0.25 and 0.5 µg capsules, Roche

Dihydrotachysterol
   Hytakerol: 0.125 mg tablet, Roche
   DHT: 0.125, 0.2, 0.4 mg tablets, 0.2 mg/ml liquid, Roxane

Calcium salts
   Various preparations and manufacturers

Appendix 3

Conversion Formulas for SI Units for Common Hormones

Hormone	SI Unit	Traditional Unit	Traditional to SI	SI to Traditional
Aldosterone	pmol/L	ng/dl	27.7	0.036
ACTH	pmol/L	pg/ml	0.22	4.51
Calcitriol	ng/L	pmol/L	2.4	0.417
Cortisol	nmol/L	μg/dl	27.59	0.36
Epinephrine	pmol/L	pg/ml	5.46	0.183
Estradiol	pmol/L	pg/ml	3.67	0.273
Insulin	pmol/L	μU/ml	7.18	0.139
17-hydroxyproges-terone	nmol/L	μg/dl	3.03	0.33
Norepinephrine	pmol/L	ng/L	5.91	0.169
Progesterone	mmol/L	ng/ml	3.18	0.315
Prolactin	pmol/L	μg/L	44.4	0.023
Testosterone	nmol/L	ng/ml	3.47	0.288
Thyroxine	nmol/L	μg/dl	12.87	0.078
Free Thyroxine	pmol/L	ng/dl	12.87	0.078
Triiodothyronine	nmol/L	ng/dl	0.0154	6.49
Vasopressin (ADH)	pg/ml	pmol/L	0.99	1.0

Appendix 4

Endocrine Testing Laboratories

Animal Health Diagnostic Laboratory
Endocrine Diagnostic Section
619 West Fee Hall B
Michigan State University
College of Veterinary Medicine
East Lansing, MI 48824-1315
(517) 353-0621

Animal Health Diagnostic Laboratory
College of Veterinary Medicine
Cornell University
Upper Tower Rd
Ithaca, NY 14853
(607) 253-3674

Clinical Endocrinology Laboratory
University of Tennessee
2407 River Dr., Rm A105, VTH
Knoxville, TN 37996
(865) 974-5638

Endocrine Diagnostic Service
Department of Physiology and Pharmacology
Auburn University College of Veterinary Medicine
Auburn, AL 36849
(334) 844-5400

Purdue University
School of Veterinary Medicine
Clinical Pathology Laboratory – Clinical Endocrinology
G351 Lynn Hall
West Lafayette, IN 47907-1249
(765) 494-3972

University of Minnesota Veterinary Diagnostic Laboratory
Endocrinology Laboratory
1333 Gortner Ave.
St. Paul, MN 55108
(612) 624-8787

Index

A

Acarbose, 172
   for diabetes mellitus, 127
Acidosis, metabolic, 132
Acromegaly
   clinical signs of
      in cats, 17
      in dogs, 18
   diagnostic imaging and tests for, 19-20
   laboratory tests for, 19
   overview of, 16-17
   prognosis for, 21
   treatment for, 20-21
ACTH. See Adrenocorticotropin (ACTH)
ACTH response test
   advantages of, 66
   with aminoglutethimide treatment, 85
   in diabetes mellitus control, 75
   in feline hyperadrenocorticism, 80
   in hyperadrenocorticism, 61-62
   in hypoglycemia, 145
   with metyrapone treatment, 84
   with mitotane treatment, 69-71
   with trilostane treatment, 85
ACTH stimulation test
   for feline hypoadrenocorticism, 97
   in hypercalcemia, 156
   for hypoadrenocorticism, 92-93
Addisonian crisis, 93
   initial treatment of, 94-95
Addison's disease. See Hypoadrenocorticism
Adrenal drugs, 172-173
Adrenal function
   in congenital growth hormone deficiency, 22
   in polyuria and polydipsia, 7
Adrenal gland

adenoma of in canine hyperadrenocorticism, 59
tumors of
   in canine hyperadrenocorticism, 58
   differentiating from pituitary-dependent hyperadrenocorticism, 66-67
   with feline hyperadrenocorticism, 77
   in hyperaldosteronism, 101
   low-dose dexamethasone suppression test in, 65
   mitotane for, 70
   surgical management of, 76
Adrenalectomy, 76
   for feline hyperadrenocorticism, 82-83
   for pheochromocytoma, 108
Adrenocortical adenoma, 54
Adrenocortical tumors, 106
Adrenocorticotropin (ACTH)
   endogenous plasma concentration of, 67-68
      in feline hyperadrenocorticism, 81-82
      in hypoadrenocorticism, 93
   excessive production of, 54
   mitotane treatment and concentrations of, 69-71
   preparations of, 173
   SI unit conversion for, 174
Adrenomegaly
   in feline hyperadrenocorticism, 79
   for hyperaldosteronism, 101
Agranulocytosis, 48
Alanine aminotransferase, 57
Aldosterone. See also Hyperaldosteronism
   deficiency of, 90
   excessive, 100, 101-102
   SI unit conversion for, 174
Alendronate, 173
Alkalosis, metabolic, 101
Alopecia
   in canine hyperadrenocorticism, 55
   in feline hyperadrenocorticism, 77, 78

Fludrocortisone, 173
    for hypoadrenocorticism, 96
Fludrocortisone acetate, 96
Fluid therapy
    for Addisonian crisis, 94
    in diabetic ketoacidosis, 134-135
    for feline hypoadrenocorticism, 98
    for hypercalcemia, 159
    for hyperparathyroidism, 161
Fructosamine, 125-126
Furosemide
    for hypercalcemia, 159
    for hypoglycemic crisis, 146

G

Galactorrhea, 29
Gallop rhythm, 41
Gastroenteritis, 155
Gastrointestinal disorders, 42
GI hemorrhage, 90, 91
Glipizide, 172
    for diabetes mellitus, 126-127
Glomerular filtration rate, 7-8
Glucagon, 172
    for hypoglycemic crisis, 146
Glucocorticoids
    for Addisonian crisis, 94-95
    deficiency of, 89
        in hypoadrenocorticism, 91, 92
    for feline hypoadrenocorticism, 98
    for hypoadrenocorticism, 96-97
    for hypoglycemic crisis, 146
    in insulin resistance, 123
    for insulinoma, 148
    preparations of, 173
Glucometers, hand-held, 144
Glucose, urine concentrations of, 125
Glucose curve, 117-124
    alternatives to, 125-126
    stress effect on, 119
Glyburide, 172

Glycosuria
    in acromegaly, 19
    in diabetes mellitus, 112
    in diabetic ketoacidosis, 133
    urinalysis for, 5
Glycosylated hemoglobin, 125-126
Growth hormone disorders, 16-23
Growth hormones, 171
    serum concentrations of, 20
Growth plates, delayed closure of, 22

H

Heart murmur, 41, 101
Hepatic failure, 143, 144
Hepatomegaly, 78, 79
Hepatopathy, 48-49
Hind limb weakness, 128
Horner's syndrome, 52
Human growth hormone, 23
Hydrocortisone, 95
25-Hydroxycholecalciferol, 159
17-Hydroxyprogesterone, SI unit
    conversion for, 174
Hyperactivity, 41
Hyperadrenocorticism
    adrenal-dependent, 54
    canine
        adrenalrenalectomy in, 76
        clinical signs of, 55-56
        diagnostic imaging for, 57-59
        discriminatory tests for, 66-68
        laboratory tests for, 57
        managing diabetes mellitus in, 75
        monitoring of, 70-74
        pituitary macroadenoma treatment
            in, 75
        problems and overview of, 54-55
        prognosis for, 76
        screening tests for, 59-66
        treatment of, 68-74
    in diabetes mellitus, 110

supportive care for, 138
treatment of, 134-139
Ketoconazole, 172
for canine hyperadrenocorticism, 73-74
for feline hyperadrenocorticism, 84
Ketone body production, 132
Ketonuria, 133

L

L-deprenyl (selegiline)
for acromegaly, 21
for canine hyperadrenocorticism, 72-73
complications and adverse drug
interactions of, 73
Laryngeal paralysis
with percutaneous ethanol injection, 51
with surgical thyroidectomy, 52
Leiomyosarcoma, 146
Levothyroxine, 171
complications of, 38
for hypothyroidism, 37
for permanent hypothyroidism, 52
therapeutic trial with in
hypothyroidism, 36
Liothyronine, 171
Liver function testing, 145
Lung aspiration, 156
Lymph nodes
aspiration/biopsy of, 156
enlargement of in hypercalcemia, 153
Lymphadenopathy, 5
Lymphosarcoma, 153

M

Magnetic resonance imaging (MRI)
for acromegaly, 19
in congenital growth hormone
deficiency, 22
Mannitol, 146
Megaesophagus
in hypoadrenocorticism, 91, 92

in hypoglycemia, 144
in hypothyroidism, 28
Metastasis, insulinoma, 148
Metformin, 172
for diabetes mellitus, 127
Methimazole, 171
complications of, 48-49
for hyperthyroidism, 47-48
Metyrapone, 173
for feline hyperadrenocorticism, 84
Mineralocorticoids, 89
deficiency of, 95
for feline hypoadrenocorticism, 98
for hypoadrenocorticism, 96-97
Mithramycin, 160
Mitotane, 172
for feline hyperadrenocorticism, 83-84
for hyperadrenocorticism, 68-69
with adrenal tumors, 70
maintenance, 71-72
monitoring, 70-71
pituitary-dependent, 69-70
Myalgia, 100
Myelinolysis, 95
Myxedema stupor, 29

N

Neurologic disorders
in hyperthyroidism, 42
in hypothyroidism, 28
Non-islet cell tumors, 143
Norepinephrine, SI unit conversion for, 174

O

Octreotide, 172
for acromegaly, 20
for insulinoma, 148
Ocular disorders, 29
Ovariohysterectomy, 20

P

Pamidronate, 173

Pamidronate disodium, 160

Pancreatectomy, 147

Pancreatic drugs, 172

Pancreatitis
   in diabetes mellitus, 129
   in hypercalcemia, 155

Parathyroid gland enlargement, 160

Parathyroid hormone (PTH)
   analysis of in hypercalcemia, 158
   elevated concentrations of, 156, 160-162
   regulated feedback loop for, 152
   serum concentration of in hypocalcemia, 166

Parathyroid hormone-related protein (PTH-RP) analysis, 158

Parathyroid mass, 154

Parathyroidectomy, 161-162

Pegvisomant, 20

Pendulous abdomen
   in canine hyperadrenocorticism, 55
   in feline hyperadrenocorticism, 77, 78

Percutaneous ethanol injection
   complications of, 51
   for hyperthyroidism, 51

Peripheral neuropathy
   in diabetes mellitus, 111, 128
   in hypothyroidism, 28

Phenoxybenzamine, 108

Pheochromocytoma
   clinical signs of, 106-107
   diagnostic imaging for, 107
   diagnostic tests for, 108
   laboratory tests for, 107
   problems and overview of, 106
   prognosis for, 108
   treatment for, 108

Phosphate supplementation, 137-138

Phosphorus
   in hypercalcemia, 156

   in hyperparathyroidism, 160

Pituitary adenoma, 54

Pituitary drugs, 171

Pituitary dwarfism. *See* Congenital growth hormone deficiency

Pituitary macroadenoma, 75

Pituitary tumor
   in acromegaly, 20
   in canine hyperadrenocorticism, 56

Plicamycin (mithramycin), 160

Pollakiuria, differentiation of, 5

Polydipsia, 4
   in canine hyperadrenocorticism, 55
   causes of, 4
   in diabetes insipidus, 11-13
   diagnostic approach to, 5-11
   in feline hyperadrenocorticism, 77
   history and physical examination for, 5
   in hyperaldosteronism, 101
   in hypercalcemia, 154
   in hyperthyroidism, 41
   laboratory tests for, 5-7
   treatment of, 13

Polyneuropathy, 28

Polyphagia
   in canine hyperadrenocorticism, 55
   in feline hyperadrenocorticism, 77
   in hyperthyroidism, 41

Polyuria, 4
   in canine hyperadrenocorticism, 55
   causes of, 4
   in diabetes insipidus, 11-13
   diagnostic approach to, 5-11
   in feline hyperadrenocorticism, 77
   history and physical examination for, 5
   in hyperaldosteronism, 101
   in hypercalcemia, 154
   in hyperthyroidism, 41
   laboratory tests for, 5-7
   treatment of, 13

Potassium chloride, 172

Potassium iodide, 171
Potassium phosphate, 172
  for diabetic ketoacidosis, 137-138
Potassium supplementation, 138
Prazosin, 108
Prednisolone, 96
Prednisone
  for cortisol deficiency, 71
  for hypercalcemia, 159
  for hypoadrenocorticism, 96-97
Progesterone
  in acromegaly, 18
  SI unit conversion for, 174
Progesterone secreting adrenal tumors, 77
Progestins, 123
Progestogen, 23
Prolactin, SI unit conversion for, 174
Propylthiouracil, 171
Proteinuria
  in acromegaly, 19
  in canine hyperadrenocorticism, 57
  in diabetes mellitus, 112
Pruritus, 27
Pyelonephritis, 5
Pyuria, 5

R

Radioactive iodine
  complications of, 51
  for hyperthyroidism, 50
Radiography
  abdominal
    for canine hyperadrenocorticism, 57
    for diabetic ketoacidosis, 134
    for hyperadrenocorticism, 68
    for pheochromocytoma, 107
  for acromegaly, 19
  for hyperaldosteronism, 101
  for hypercalcemia, 157
  for hypoadrenocorticism, 92
  for hypothyroidism, 30

thoracic
  for canine hyperadrenocorticism, 58
  for diabetic ketoacidosis, 134
  for hyperthyroidism, 43
  for pheochromocytoma, 107
Renal failure
  in acromegaly, 19
  evidence of, 5
  in hypercalcemia, 153, 154
Renal function, 48
Renal imaging, 7
Reproductive disorders, 29
Retinal hemorrhage, 101
Retinopathy
  in diabetes mellitus, 129
  hypertensive, 42, 101

S

Salt supplementation, 97
Scintigraphy with metaiodobenzylguanidine (MIBG), 108
Seizures
  emergency treatment of, 166-167
  in hypercalcemia, 155
  in hypocalcemia, 165
Selegiline
  for acromegaly, 21
  adverse drug interactions of, 73
  for canine hyperadrenocorticism, 72-73
Sepsis, 144
Serum chemistries
  in hypercalcemia, 155-156
  in hyperthyroidism, 43
  in hypoglycemia, 143
  in polyuria and polydipsia, 6
SI units, conversion formulas for, 174
Sodium bicarbonate
  for diabetic ketoacidosis, 137
  for hypercalcemia, 159
Soft tissue mineralization, 154
Somatostatin analog

Urinalysis
  for diabetes mellitus, 126
  in hypercalcemia, 156
  in hyperthyroidism, 43
  in hypoglycemia, 143
  for polyuria and polydipsia, 5
Urinary tract infection
  in canine hyperadrenocorticism, 57
  in diabetes insipidus, 12
  in diabetes mellitus, 112, 129
  in hypercalcemia, 154, 156
  in hyperparathyroidism, 160
  in insulin resistance, 124
Urine
  glucose levels in, 125
  ketones in, 139-140
  specific gravity of in diabetes insipidus, 12
Urine cortisol: creatinine ratio
  in feline hyperadrenocorticism, 79-80
  in hyperadrenocorticism, 60-61
  with L-deprenyl treatment, 72
Urine culture
  in canine hyperadrenocorticism, 57
  in diabetes mellitus, 112
  in diabetic ketoacidosis, 133
  for polyuria and polydipsia, 5
Urolithiasis, 160

V

Vanadium, 127
Vasopressin
  preparations of, 171
  SI unit conversion for, 174
Venipuncture, 118
Venography, 107
Vetsulin, 172
Vitamin D
  for hypercalcemia, 153
  for hypocalcemia, 164
  for hypoparathyroidism, 169
  for non-emergent hypocalcemia, 167-168

  for postoperative hypocalcemia, 162
Vitamin D toxicity
  in hypercalcemia, 159
  treatment of, 160
Vomiting, 48

W

Water deprivation test
  for diabetes insipidus, 12
  in polyuria and polydipsia, 8-10
Water intake
  in diabetes insipidus, 13
  in polydipsia, 5
Weight loss
  for diabetes mellitus, 115
  in hyperthyroidism, 40

X

Xylazine, 22